The
Beginning
of
Everything

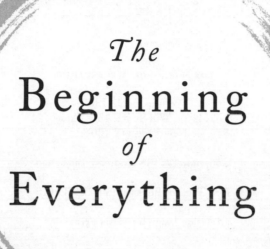

The
Beginning
of
Everything

Andrea J. Buchanan

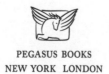

PEGASUS BOOKS
NEW YORK LONDON

THE BEGINNING OF EVERYTHING

Pegasus Books Ltd.
148 W. 37th Street, 13th Floor
New York, NY 10018

Copyright © 2018 Andrea J. Buchanan

First Pegasus Books edition April 2018

Interior design by Maria Fernandez

Library of Congress Cataloging-in-Publication Data is available.

ISBN: 978-1-68177-672-9

10 9 8 7 6 5 4 3 2 1

Printed in the United States of America
Distributed by W. W. Norton & Company

To Emi and Nate

Contents

Introduction

I lost my mind on the way to brunch one particularly bitter Sunday in March of 2015. It is a moment I return to over and over again: the wind biting at my face, my body sweaty with fever, my throat fiery with virus as I crossed the street, inhaled that March wind, and choked on it.

There was a lot I was choking on that day. Sending my kids off for the weekend with their father, even though my son had woken up with a 103-degree fever, his face pink, curls filigreed to his cheeks and forehead. The dread of my own fever aching through me as I began sinking into sickness myself. The knot in my stomach of my divorce, the fighting and lawyering, a seemingly endless battle. The guilt of failing, as a partner, as a mother.

And so I coughed as the wind sucked itself into me, lodging itself in my throat. I doubled over in the midst of the intersection, unable to escape the chokehold of the vicious tickle I couldn't displace. At the time, my worry was that I would vomit on the street due to the cough's intensity, and I remember feeling relieved when I was finally able to breathe again, to drink some water, to talk without my throat seizing up. I thought it was over.

I couldn't have been more wrong.

Because when I stood hunched over in the wind in the middle of the street, I also stood in the middle of a perfect confluence of events. Because when I coughed and coughed the wind out of my throat that day, when I choked on everything that was choking me that day, I also, somehow, ripped a small tear in my dura mater, the tough membrane covering my brain and spinal cord. But I didn't know that yet. Instead, I crossed the street, wiped away the tears running down my face from the wind, walked to the restaurant with my friend and drank water and shivered through my fever and ate French toast, all completely unaware that at that moment, my cerebrospinal fluid was already beginning to leak out of the tiny, jagged tear somewhere along my thoracic spine.

What followed was nine months of intractable pain and the inability to be upright for more than minutes at a time. A constant ache at the back of my head as my brain, no longer cushioned by a healthy waterbed of fluid, sank to the bottom of my skull. A confusion of neurological symptoms, of brain fog and cognitive impairment to the point where I couldn't think, couldn't write, couldn't follow instructions or watch television or hold conversations or make sense of even the most basic concepts. At a time in my life when I needed to be as independent and autonomous and clear-thinking as possible—in the midst of a divorce after twenty years of marriage, with two teenaged children to shepherd through the upheaval of their lives and everything they'd come to depend on—I was trapped by my brain, stuck in bed, unable to do anything more than lie flat and stare at the ceiling and hope for sleep to edge out the pain that had become the defining characteristic of my consciousness.

My diagnosis of spontaneous intracranial hypotension confounded the doctors I saw, none of whom could agree on where, precisely, this "brain leak," as one of them had called it, might be located, or how to cure it. I floated through the fog from one specialist to another, enduring skepticism and condescension and strange, barbaric-seeming procedures, before finally arriving in North Carolina, at Duke University, where a team of neuroradiologists immediately recognized my constellation of symptoms and set about fixing me.

As I began the long, slow process of recovery, and as my brain slowly began to return to me, finally cushioned by enough cerebrospinal fluid to float the way it should, all those cramped and squashed nerves stretching back to their previous form, I had a lot of time to think about what had happened. While it was happening, of course, I had only fleeting moments of lucidity: My world, during the leak, was pain, fog, uncertainty, frustration; but I couldn't think much deeper than that. As I began to heal, I realized that my brain's inability to function at any level other than the most basic had, ironically, helped me keep going during that time, as the existential terror of it all only began to fully sink in once I was able to think again.

I kept trying to find ways to understand it, to go back in time and prevent it, to give it a narrative that made sense. All the stories I told myself were bound up in blame, in guilt, in personal culpability. Even though I recognized how powerless I was to control any of it—the tear in my dura, the regulation of my CSF fluid, the sinking of my brain—in the foggy chain of events I invented to explain myself, the only thing that made sense was some deficiency on my part, some simple thing I could have done, or not done, if only I'd been better, smarter, somehow more deserving. For surely I must have deserved this, it couldn't be a mere accident that this accident happened now, in the midst of my ripping apart my family for something as insignificant and self-indulgent as my own happiness.

And yet even my still-foggy brain, desperate for puzzle pieces that soothingly, predictably fit together, was aware of the fundamental self-indulgence of that narrative, and the ultimate futility of trying to trace back the source. What good would it do to understand the precise nature of the moment my body tore in some mysterious spot? Would it make me tougher once I realized the fragility of my own choices? Even if I could pinpoint the inciting incident, could absolving myself of the guilt knit up the frayed edges of my dura mater, fix me, heal me, make me a good mother?

These thoughts were largely too large to grapple with in my still-foggy state. In hopeless moments of clarity, they would float to the surface, along with worries about how I would work if I never fully recovered, how I would survive making dinner for the kids that night, how I would live the rest of my life if it was going to be like this forever, and I would promptly fall asleep, the pain in my head a flat constant warning buzz, my brain too overwhelmed to think about itself any longer.

But as my brain continued to heal, and as I began to find myself less trapped in my bed and more a commuter between the two worlds of the sick and the well, I found myself drawn to stories. True stories about science's search for understanding of the brain's capacity to heal itself; stories of early, technology-deprived adventurers pushing the brain to its limits in the thin air of Everest; the modern spiritual folktales of "mind over matter," "thinking positive," and "brain training"; the ancient tropes of fairy tales, making meaning out of suffering, solitude, and transformation. I wanted to know: Where was "I" when I wasn't there? Who was I when I wasn't "myself"? And who was I when I couldn't think? The more

I recovered, the more I was able to contemplate these questions, and eventually—gradually, slowly—I began to trust that it was, if not exactly safe to start depending on my brain again, important to reconnect myself to the world as surely as the pathways in my brain reconnected themselves. To get on with the ongoing business of living, which had never waited for me to catch up to it. To stop dreading the seemingly inevitable return of the pain and fog, the clouding of my brain no medical professional could assure me with 100 percent certainty would never happen again. I found myself instead on the other side of the divide: divorced, instead of divorcing; healing, while being mindful of the time I spent unwell. The questions of self and agency and autonomy still haunt me, even as now I have begun to move through the world again and take everything for granted. But I have come to understand that, whether or not the leak returns, whether or not the me that is me is truly the me I understand it to be—this is who I am. A woman standing, leaning into the wind, just like that cold day in March, in the midst of my life, in the middle of an intersection of body and mind and circumstance and history, and maybe even fate.

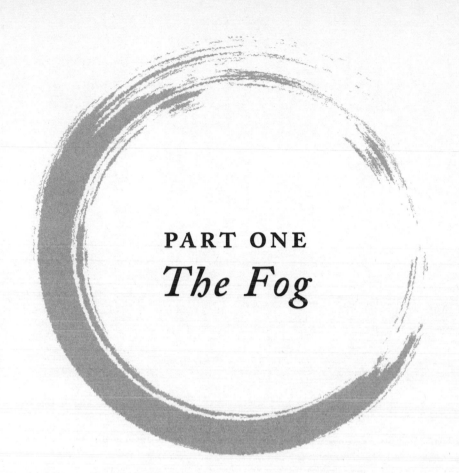

PART ONE
The Fog

Spontaneous intracranial hypotension is an uncommon but not rare cause of new onset daily persistent headaches. A delay in diagnosis is the norm. Women are affected more commonly than men and most are in the fifth or sixth decade of life. The underlying cause is a spontaneous spinal cerebrospinal fluid (CSF) leak. Typically the headache is orthostatic in nature but other headache patterns occur as well. Associated symptoms are common and include neck pain, a change in hearing, diplopia, facial numbness, cognitive abnormalities and even coma. Typical imaging findings consist of subdural fluid collections, pachymeningeal enhancement, pituitary hyperaemia and brain sagging, but magnetic resonance imaging may be normal. Myelography is the study of choice to identify the CSF leak but is not always necessary to make the diagnosis. Treatment consists of bedrest, abdominal binder, epidural blood patching, percutaneous fibrin glue injection or surgical CSF leak repair. Outcomes have been poorly studied.

—Wouter I. Schievink,
"Spontaneous spinal cerebrospinal fluid leaks,"
Cephalalgia, 2008

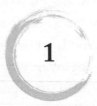

1

I am an unreliable narrator.

 And yet, here in the doctor's office, it is required of me to tell my story.

Where does it hurt? Does the pain change? When did this start?

These are valid questions, but attempting to answer them, attempting to explain from the inside out, seems impossible. At first because the pain is so distracting, a softball-sized hit to the base of my skull, my hands perpetually massaging it at the back of my head, as though it could be possible to ease it out physically, if only my fingers were strong enough.

 And then because, after a time, after so much constant pain, it becomes impossible to think at all. Words float away from me, simple questions cloak themselves in impenetrable meaning, I find myself lost in the long pauses I find compulsory to take when answering things like "How long do the headaches last?" or "How many days a month do you have a headache?" or "When did this start?"

And then of course because my narration is suspect. You will have to believe me when I say that it is hard for me to be believed, that I say "headache" and the doctor writes down "migraine," even though I have no history of migraine; that I describe my symptoms and am asked, a knowing nod, an eyebrow raised, "How old are you again, 43?"; that I present my history and find myself met with skepticism about the veracity of my reporting.

Have you tried ibuprofen? Have you tried caffeine? Have you tried meditation? Deep breathing? Vitamin D?

What they are really asking is, *Have you tried not being a 43-year-old woman in the midst of a divorce?*

It's a headache, I'm a woman. How is this a mystery?

"When did this start?" is the hardest question to answer. It should be the easiest, because how else do you start telling a story except at the beginning? I see now the advantage of fairy tales, of the old stories that begin in the far-off haze of "Once upon a time," because who can say definitively when the start of anything was? When the earth cooled? When the universe was born? Trying to find the inciting event is like trying to trace back the decay of my marriage: Was there even a starting point? Is there one specific, defining moment in time I can point to and understand, yes, that was it, that was where it fell apart, that was the moment everything became inevitable? Or is it more cumulative, small moments snowballing into a cascade of insurmountable differences? And if it's that, then would it have even been possible to stop it, to catch one hurtling snowball of a moment and thus prevent the avalanche? Could I have saved myself from either of these things?

"When did it start?" is the hardest question to answer, because I don't even know what *it* is.

I could say March 21, 2015, around 10:30 A.M., because that's when I had the coughing fit.

I could say about a week after that, because that's when I first started to realize that the sneaking, nagging headache was becoming something constant and unrelenting.

But I could also say any moment of any day of any year.

The day I sat at the keys of a concert grand, my ten-year-old hands frozen for a moment as the audience waited expectantly, my pedal foot shaking, my heart racing, my mind, for a terrible moment, entirely blank just before the second I closed my eyes and my fingers began playing the sonata that I was sure, up until then, I couldn't remember. The day I walked by myself at night, in the Boston winter, as a teenager, and was followed into a store by a man who lingered, shadowing me, until I whispered tearfully to a kindly clerk, who kicked him out and escorted me home. The day my first ever piano was delivered to me, my engagement ring, a gift from my husband-to-be, the sun streaming through the skylights of our loft, and me standing there, thinking *How do I deserve this?* The day I held my newborn daughter, her drowsy baby breath in my ear still catching on hiccupy sobs as I paced the hallway of our apartment, bouncing with every step, patting her gently, easing her into sleep. The day I cried so hard after a fight with my husband, my eyes puffed shut. The day I walked off a bus and into a hailstorm, ice pellets hitting me, leaving round purple-green marks I would only discover days later, ghosts of the storm. The day I slept off a fever. The day I pushed myself through a fever. The day I was born. The day, months before I was born, when the thick membrane covering my spinal cord and brain was formed, the connective tissue connecting itself, but only thinly in this one small place that might not even matter unless I one day had a fever, left the house, went to breakfast, coughed. The day some secret was whispered to my body, the time bomb placed, the disgruntled fairy's curse destined to come to pass, no matter how many spinning wheels are burned, no matter what steps are taken to avoid it. Any of these days could have been the day this all started, that this burgeoning thing inside me swelled, that my cerebrospinal fluid surged and my dura strained and the one thin spot became thinner, until the day it thinned so precisely it was possible for the truth to leak out.

Not everything is an epiphany. You can't always know the precise moment you fall in love, or out of love, or when the creeping sensation you feel becomes a solid, present pain. Things happen in aggregate, they accrete. Signs accumulate until suddenly it is impossible to not see them as anything except inevitable, omnipresent. They have somehow, suddenly, always existed.

And yet I recognize this impulse, this tracing and retracing, this quest to make reliable my unreliable narration, as a way to locate this within me, literally within me, within my control, and thus within my power to change it.

I cannot change it.

"When did this start?" is the hardest question to answer, because of how it is twinned for me with its ghost question: *What did you do to cause this?* And the answer to that is that I coughed, and also that I had a fever, and also that I fell out of love, and also that I became unhappy, and also that I wasn't able to overcome my unhappiness, and also that I wasn't able to save my marriage, and also that I failed, and so when I try to answer the question "When did this start?" I am also trying to answer the questions *How did I let this happen?* and *Why couldn't I just be happy?* and *What can I do to undo this?* and *If I think hard enough to find my way back to the beginning, will that be enough to break the spell, undo this curse, right this wrong, make everything whole again?*

"When did this start?" the doctor asks, and I say, "March, probably March, end of March."

2

There are a lot of things you can do, it turns out, while leaking cerebrospinal fluid.

You can take a fifteen-year-old to a Twitter meet-up of fifty Ariana Grande fans, as long as you find a comfortable chair in the hotel lobby and slump down as far as you can to be as close to horizontal as possible, waving off the other parents with vague excuses about a migraine, even though it's not a migraine, because that seems the quickest way to get people to both understand and to leave you alone, clutching the back of your head where a lump of pain has taken over the back right base of your skull.

You can serve on a jury, as long as you will yourself to not lie down on the courtroom floor, even though you mentioned to the judge that you had a something like a migraine, but that wasn't enough to excuse you, and so it turns out you can sit up and hold the back of your head and listen to a very new lawyer extract relevant info from his very clueless client, who seems so unfamiliar with the details of his own case it seems possible that he, too, might be leaking cerebrospinal fluid, and then eat a tuna sandwich with the other jurors and find for the defendant.

A few weeks after that, you can agree with your husband that it's time to tell your kids that you are getting divorced, even though by this point you can't really sit up anymore, because being upright brings on the relentless back-of-skull headache, and even when you lie flat in bed the world seems tipsy, you feel tipsy, that sense of drunken confidence flooding you even as you're aware you might not be saying things the way you meant to, and you can't not cry when your daughter turns away and starts texting her friends, when you ask your son if he has any questions and he says "Yes. Can you not get divorced?", when your head hurts so much the pain is all you have room for and you can't absorb theirs the way you'd planned to before, when your brain was all yours.

You can do things like this because at this point you don't know you're leaking cerebrospinal fluid, you don't fully know what's going on, and you have yet to realize what a problem that is, because the thing you use to think with is the very thing that's problematic.

The problem you have, when you have a problem with your brain, is that your brain doesn't necessarily realize that it's having a problem. It keeps trying to strategize, rationalize, keep you in motion. It keeps supplying you with ideas, convincing you with plausible excuses, explanations. Like: *You're fine! See how normal you feel when you stay completely still and flat and close your eyes and don't move? Just keep doing that!* Or: *People have headaches all the time! Go ahead and cook dinner, just take breaks by lying on the floor, that's a smart solution! You got this!*

But you're not thinking, exactly. You're in a fog, and all the time you're floating on the surface of things, you're padded, your real self stuck inside this swollen busy-work instructive primal machine that's taken over to keep you moving, and ideas float to you from somewhere and your uncushioned brain just says, *Yes, it makes sense to lie down here in the middle of the kitchen floor while you wait for the timer to go off so you can stand up and drain the pasta and then lie down again for a few moments before you have to add the sauce, that's normal.* Your brain says, *It's okay, remember, this is just a thing that happens now, like how when you lie down and close your eyes you can't feel your arms anymore.* Your brain tells you, *It's fine to be curled up here in the chair unable to open your eyes while these five doctors talk at you, just nod your head, they deal with sick people all the time, you're probably not being rude,* while the experts are telling you "Your call, you decide" whether or not to be admitted to the hospital, to have surgery, to stay home, to wait it out. And all along your brain is doggedly continuing to try to make sense of it all, the way it does in a dream, the way dream logic seems so right until you wake up.

When exactly do I wake up?

3

I n the doctor's offices, I recite my history like an incantation. There is a rhythm to it now, like an ancient spell, and I have learned the True Speak of the medical wizards: I know which terms will unlock the vaults of understanding, which magical words—*orthostatic, occipital*—will make visible the thing I am conjuring, what syllables can transform me from a tired rambling woman into a wise witch, full of insight and secrets that could explain everything if they only listened true.

There is the truth of my experience, and the truth of the doctors' diagnostic limitations. Even with machines they cannot see the small tear in the fabric of my reality. And yet my descriptions of what it feels like to lose my brain from the inside out are irrelevant to them, despite being the only thing relevant to me, the entirety of my comprehension. Everything is pain and confusion.

They speak in riddles, though I am aware there is no trickery intended. It is my brain, fluid-deprived and desperate, attempting to understand even the simplest of questions. I have always previously had the luxury of this being an unconscious, painless process. But now it is a trial. A prick of the finger on a spinning wheel, a hero's journey, a boulder pushed up a mountain.

There are things I can say without thinking. My mouth opens and words come out, free-associated comments I am often only able to make half-sense of afterward, trying to cover my confusion with humor. I am able to fool some people; they aren't able to sense my panic, my terror at not knowing who is speaking when I hear myself talking out loud.

In the doctor's offices I rely on the magic words I have learned in order to be taken seriously—*sudden onset* and *no history of migraine*, and, crucially, *positional*—and I repeat them, when I am asked, and the doctors nod at me and scribble, or type at a computer, and sometimes I am buoyed by the way they seem to be listening, and I tell my story with all the rich details I can muster, hoping that with my words I can convince them of the pain and terror and confusion they cannot see and cannot trace and even with their powers cannot fix. More often, though, I lie flat, staring into the fluorescent lights, lost in the patterns on the ceiling, the stains and crevices, tears choking my voice as I whisper whatever facts I can muster in response to whatever questions they ask.

Are these sorcerer's riddles? Must I answer by not answering, is that the trick, to instead somehow divine by holy inspiration the correct response so as to earn my passage through the wizard's vale? Each appointment is a quest I must complete as I hover in the mist, all things obscured.

4

April 2015

It takes me centuries to get dressed. I pause for eons in front of the mirror as I try to remember why I'm bothering to brush my hair. I blink, and when I open my eyes time has passed, enough for new universes to be born, enough for the sun to have burned out, imploded, the world gone. Somehow I am clothed, am downstairs, am ready to go. I blink and I'm in a cab, lying down in the backseat, jostled, gauging the route by how many turns I feel the car making. Blink again and I am sitting up, credit card in hand, confounded by the payment machine. Blink again and I am outside the hospital, upright, wincing in the sun. Blink again and I am upstairs, in the neuro-ophthalmology department, sitting

14

in a chair, confronted by a form. So many boxes, so many lines, so many questions. Name, birthday, address, insurance. I write what I can remember and find a corner of the waiting area. I lie down.

Blink and I am called by a nurse. Weighed, measured. Asked why I'm there. Blood pressure high. I apologize, "My arm gets claustrophobic," I say to the nurse. She regards me with an eyebrow. Blink and I am back in the waiting area, on the floor, the nubby carpet thin and rough. There are people sitting all around me, in chairs, like they're supposed to, but I don't care. My eyes are closed. I can't see them looking at me, wondering why on earth a person would be so rude as to lie on the floor.

Blink and I am summoned by a doctor, who seems bemused as I rise out of the depths, emerging from the waiting room floor. I'm escorted to a room with an eye doctor chair, and I ask if it can be adjusted to be flat, just for a little while, but maybe he doesn't hear me. I curl up on the base of the chair, lying sideways, an awkward fetal position.

Blink and the real doctor comes in. He is a colleague of my husband's; I have encountered him for years at social events, informal pool parties and fancy dinners where I play the part of doctor-wife and make small talk while supervising my children or pretending to be a person who eats fancy dinners all the time. I have talked to him about books, about his idea for a book he wants to write. I have met his family. He knows me as a person who can sit up and have conversations. And so he is concerned to see me struggling to not slide off the chair, to watch me struggle to make sense of his questions, to witness me in pain attempting to sit up for his exam. He doesn't know about the divorce yet, none of Gil's colleagues do. He asks after Gil, who is away at a conference. I tell him Gil is fine, that he's away at a conference.

He asks what's going on, and I tell him what I know so far: that I had a terrible flu, and then a headache that wouldn't go away;

that I was given antibiotics for a suspected sinus infection, but the headache persisted. That it improves a little when I lie down, but being upright for more than five minutes brings the headache to full force, and having to be upright for more than an hour, even if I'm just sitting, not moving, basically wrecks me. Can't think clearly. So much pain.

He tells me what he suspects, based on the MRI, based on his exam. This is spontaneous intracranial hypotension, otherwise known as a spontaneous CSF leak, possibly located in my ethmoid sinus, at least according to what the radiologist saw on my MRI. Had I coughed when I had the flu? Right. Well, that could have caused a tear, or some sort of rupture. And this spot in my ethmoid sinus could be allowing cerebrospinal fluid to escape. "So what you're saying is, this is all in my head," I joke, but he answers me seriously, telling me that it's possible the suspicious area seen on the MRI could just be a totally normal thing for me, the way my anatomy has always been, and the leak could be someplace else, not in my head at all. But that's why he wants me to consult with an ENT, who is the only doctor at the hospital who deals with CSF leaks. He will evaluate me and look at my scans and maybe order more, and then we'll go from there. If it's really that area in the ethmoid sinus that's causing the leak, he says the ENT can go in through my nose and get to my brain and place some sort of mesh over the leaky spot to patch things up.

"The other thing we can do," he tells me, "is kind of a 'voodoo' procedure. It's called a blood patch. No one really knows how it works, but it sometimes works for these things. It's like having an epidural—you had an epidural with your kids, right? It's like that, but you get injected with your own blood."

This sounds horrible, so I just nod and close my eyes and sink down in the chair. I blink and there are residents in the room now, doctors in training who don't know me but know my husband. The doctor is concerned. He tells me he is considering admitting me to the hospital for the weekend, he's never seen me like this. He asks me, "Do you want to be admitted? It's your call." I don't know how to answer this. It seems like such an imposition. And what about the kids? "If I send you home, can someone take care of you, can you just lie flat for a couple of days straight, is there someone who can watch the kids?" These are all impossible questions to answer. "Can your husband take care of you?" he asks again, smiling, but I'm not smiling. I say, "Maybe if you write a prescription for that," and he pauses for a moment and then says, tactfully, "Well, that's for you guys to work out. But I'll give him a call and fill him in on things from here."

He's hesitant to send me home, but he also keeps telling me it's my call to be admitted to the hospital or not, and I can't make the decision. Eventually I blink and I am walking back into the waiting area, finding my way to the elevator bank. *Were the hallways this long when I came here this morning?* I blink and I am walking out of the elevator. I see empty couches in the mezzanine and I lie down. My head is hurting so much I can't think. I rest there for 30 minutes, 45 minutes, one eye open as I text Gil to let him know the appointment went okay, that I need to see an ENT, that his colleague thinks this is a CSF leak, that I'm supposed to be in bed for the next 72 hours, drinking lots of caffeine for some reason.

I blink and I am outside in the blinding sunlight. Blink and I am on the sidewalk near a line of cabs. Blink and I am jostling, prone, in the backseat. Blink and I am putting the key in the lock, home, lying down on the couch to assuage the pain in my head until I can make it upstairs to my bed, where I am to stay flat, doctor's orders, through the weekend.

5

Spontaneous is a funny word. Even in the context of the phrase "spontaneous cerebrospinal fluid leak," the word sounds like such a happy thing, the kind of state of mind happy people always urge people like me to embrace. I hear "spontaneous" and I think jazz hands, last-minute concert tickets, manic pixie dream plans. Well, I did it, happy people. I got spontaneous. Or at least my body did.

That cough. I'd coughed the kind of cough where you can't stop coughing, and people on the street stop to look at you bending over with the cough, trying not to vomit from coughing so much. I didn't think anything of it at the time, except how embarrassed I'd be if I actually threw up right there, mid-crosswalk, on the way to breakfast; I just eventually managed to stop coughing, and I didn't connect the dots to the headache that seeped in afterwards until now, when the doctors asked me if I'd experienced any trauma, an accident, even a really bad cough.

The neuro-ophthalmologist said that until they figure out what to do, I should lie down, and I should try to drink as much caffeine as possible—two things at which I naturally excel. So I'm doing that.

I listen to podcasts, play easy puzzle games on my phone; sometimes I listen to podcasts while playing easy puzzle games on my phone. The stories keep me company, even when I don't have the attention span to follow them. I'll drift off in the midst of nineteenth-century warfare and wake up to the technology of World War I; sleep in the middle of a talk about early twentieth-century American medicine and wake to a roundtable discussion of physics among speakers so British I can hear them stirring their tea.

It's hard not to go back in time, hard not to retrace my steps. I keep thinking: *If I'd just stayed home that weekend.* But more than that: *If I'd let them stay home that weekend.* It would have been so easy to cancel my plans, to have my kids cancel theirs with their dad. Nate was already feverish when they packed up the car, and I'd felt it myself, the tickle in my throat, the prickle of fever on my skin, the beginnings. But I ignored it, sent them off with Advil, Tylenol, the thermometer, and my goodbyes. If I hadn't, I could have taken care of him. We could have been sick together. I wouldn't have gone out for breakfast, I wouldn't have caught the wind in my throat and coughed so hard I sprung a leak. I might never have had a leak at all, because in the scenario where I would cancel my weekend plans to take care of a sick kid instead of making his dad do it, I wouldn't have been selfish.

A part of me worries that this is actually true, that it could actually work like that, that spontaneous CSF leaks happen only to selfish people, that it is my fault, that everything is my fault, that if I could have just stayed happy and stayed okay and stayed in this marriage, then I wouldn't be trapped in my head right now, anxious and terrified about what's wrong, thinking endlessly about how I could have caused it, about how frustrating it is that even though it's serious and real it's still invisible to the doctors and they don't know how to treat it, other than with bed rest and caffeine and a procedure one of the doctors openly referred to as "voodoo."

But maybe this is a thing inside me that just happened to have happened, something that would have happened eventually anyway, something that could have been triggered at any time: doing headstands in yoga class, riding roller coasters, whipping my hair out of my face, being jostled by potholes in taxis or buses. Maybe it could have happened later, after the divorce was final, after I was off the good insurance. Maybe it's for the best that it happened when it did.

This is what I mean, about my brain. Still desperately working to come up with reasons, with theories, with a narrative that makes sense, even as I lie in bed, grappling with the sensations: the draining feeling, like gravity is sucking my brain down when I try to sit up; the scraping feeling, like I'm banging around the bottom of a rusty barrel.

6

April 2015

I am back at the hospital for a consult with the ear, nose, and throat surgeon. I have spent the last three days flat, as instructed by the neuro-ophthalmologist, getting up only to use the bathroom, otherwise remaining in bed, on my back, drifting in the pain. I have tried to read about CSF leaks online, on my phone, holding it directly over my head as I lie flat, and have only discovered terrifying things. Worst-case scenario case studies in medical journals. Frantic, heartbreaking posts on message boards. I ask the physician assistant who leads me into the exam room if she can lower the chair back, whether it can be extended into something resembling a table, and she obliges, allowing me to be flat as I am asked yet again to recount my history.

When the ENT comes in, I recognize him. Not because I know him, or because he is a colleague of Gil's, but because he is the kind of doctor I have encountered before. Skeptical. Suspicious. Dismissive, with the kind of surgeon's bluster and confidence that edges on contempt for the patient. I am the patient.

"So, you think you have a CSF leak," he says, and though I am lying down at this point and can't actually see his face, the way he says the word *think* implies the eye roll he may have actually performed. I turn my head toward him as he walks to my side, extending his hand to shake mine as he introduces himself.

"I've been told that I might have a CSF leak, yes," I reply, and he nods his head. He has a kind of *gotcha!* smirk on his face as he leans closer to me, and asks, "Then why are you lying down?"

I'm confused by this question, by his hostile energy, and for a moment I can't even begin to answer. Lying down is the only thing that helps the pain even a little bit. Lying down is what a team of doctors literally just told me to do three days ago. Lying down is the only way I can manage to think, and even then just barely. I feel as though he's interrogating me like I'm on the witness stand, like he's trapped me in a lie, like he's just enacted the big prosecutorial reveal and now the gavel will sound, curtailing the shocked murmurs from the gallery, and the case will be dismissed.

"Lying down makes it hurt less," I say, trying to make it sound like a statement, not a question, and he chuckles, shaking his head, and tells me, "Get up."

Later I would learn that there are different kinds of CSF leaks, and that mine was not the kind this doctor was skilled in treating. Later I would learn that skull-based CSF leaks—like, for instance, a leak located in a person's ethmoid sinus, as the doctors suspected with me at this point—present differently than spinal CSF leaks, and never cause intracranial hypotension. With spinal CSF leaks, where a person is leaking from somewhere along the spine, lying down does indeed ameliorate some of the symptoms. But when a person with a cranial or skull-based leak lies down, cerebrospinal fluid can leak out through the nasal passages. And so for those kinds of leaks, being upright is ideal: The pressure in the head is negative, and therefore no fluid leaks from the nose. From this doctor's perspective—a doctor who had only ever encountered skull-based CSF leaks—I was a malingerer of some kind, perhaps an attention-seeker, and, either way, foolish enough to fail his test. I felt better lying down? Not proof that I might have a spinal CSF leak: Proof that I was faking.

And yet I did feel better lying down. Lying down was the only thing that brought me even slight relief. "Come on, get up," he said, and I struggled to sit up, struggled to explain that being upright made everything worse for me, and just at that moment, Gil came in. His hospital ID badge identifying him as an attending physician may as well have been a shining sword pulled from a stone, as immediately the ENT's attitude changed from skepticism to deference. I listened to them discuss me as I lay back down again, hearing the ENT's responses change from accusatory to something resembling professional interest, hearing my symptoms presented in third person, in doctor-speak, as I lay on the table, searching for patterns in the pocked ceiling.

I am asked to sit up again, nicely this time; asked to lean forward, asked to try to produce cerebrospinal fluid from my nose. "I've never leaked anything out of my nose," I tell the doctor. "I just have a terrible headache." But he urges me to try. Sitting forward, bending forward, leaning over, the pain is excruciating, and after a few minutes I can't go on any longer, I'm crying from the pain. The physician assistant sprays something in my nostrils, and the ENT examines, and they try to get me to lean over again, to leak fluid. If they can get a sample, they can test it to see if it's really cerebrospinal fluid; it will help determine if this is really a CSF leak. I lean over for a moment, but it's awful, and I'm grateful to hear Gil step in, to hear the irritation in his voice as he tells the ENT it's too much, it's not going to happen, I'm in too much pain to keep sitting in that position. I lie back down, everything pain now, and hear them discuss things in doctor tones as they peer at the computer screen showing my MRI, the notes from my primary care doctor and the neuro-ophthalmologist. Soon they return to my bedside, and there is a plan. I should have a consult with a neurosurgeon in a few days. Next Monday I will have another MRI, this time focused on the orbits, and also a CT scan of my head and neck. Tuesday I will check in with the ENT. And then Thursday I will be scheduled for through-the-face brain surgery.

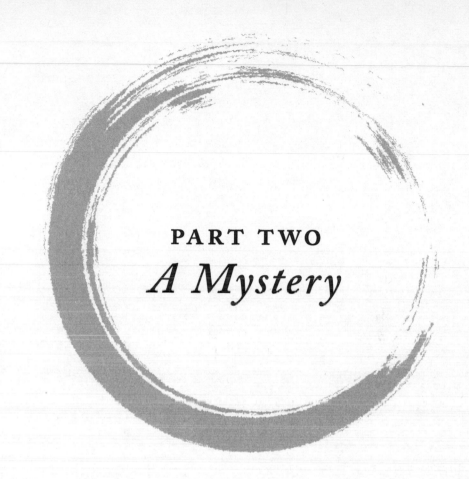

PART TWO

A Mystery

A patient presents with a new headache that occurs shortly after assuming an upright position and is relieved by lying down. Although such a positional headache pattern is well-known following a diagnostic lumbar puncture, the spontaneous onset of an orthostatic headache is not well recognized and the patient may be diagnosed with migraine, tension headache, viral meningitis, or malingering. This has been a typical scenario for many patients experiencing spontaneous intracranial hypotension . . . [and] an initial misdiagnosis remains the norm. Unfamiliarity with spontaneous intracranial hypotension among physicians in general and the unusually varied spectrum of clinical and radiographic manifestations may all contribute to a delay in diagnosis that often is measured in months or even years and decades.

—Wouter I. Schievink,
"Spontaneous Spinal Cerebrospinal Fluid Leaks and Intracranial Hypotension," *JAMA*, 2006

7

The days pass by in a series of blinks and I fumble my way through an appointment with a neurosurgeon the ENT suggested I see. My sister drives me, lets me lie down in her car, helps me joke about my weird leaking brain. The neurosurgeon listens to my now rote recitation of my history, thumbs the file from the ENT, and says sure, this probably really is a CSF leak, and says sure, the through-the-face surgery to fix it is probably fine—if that's really where the leak is. If not, the surgery could actually cause a new leak, and there's also a significant risk of my losing my ability to smell. But it's up to me. My call.

I blink and then I am somehow back at the hospital, waiting for the next MRI and CT, a nurse taking pity on me and allowing me to lie in a free bed while I wait for the CT, while they insert the IV I need for the MRI, while they fix it after it fills with blood. I'm given powerful antibiotics in advance of the through-the-face surgery that it is my call to have done. It is some kind of fluoroquinolone, and I take only one pill before I notice my previously injured ankle tendon feeling strange, and then google to see if that could somehow be a kind of side effect and discover a host of warnings about the dangers and risks of fluoroquinolones (including tendon problems), and I stop taking it.

I blink and days later there is a flurry of activity, sudden phone calls and intense consultations, when the CT scan of my neck is shown to have revealed a secret fracture—an old injury to the second cervical vertebra. The first vertebra, C1, is where the skull attaches to the neck. The C2 vertebra, sometimes called the axis vertebra, allows the head to rotate. It is actually connected to C1 by a tooth-like protuberance called the dens, and it is this, the dens, that has appeared on my CT scan as damaged, fractured somehow, long ago. Looking up information about this anatomy, I'm pleased to read that the C2 and its toothy dens has a rare nickname: vertebra dentata. There is concern, however, that this fracture may be the source of my leak, that this vertebra dentata has in fact somehow chewed through my dura. But this seems unlikely to the ENT; he is more concerned with the shadowy spot around my ethmoid sinus. He recommends further CTs and X-rays of this old C2 fracture, a consultation with yet another neurosurgeon, all things that can be done after my surgery.

I show up the day of surgery and go through the motions of filling out forms, being checked in. Gil is there this time, and he handles the things that are too complicated, answering questions for me, doing the paperwork. I'm able to lie flat on a bed in the pre-op area, and this is a relief. I'm told the surgery will involve first pumping some glow-in-the-dark stuff up through my spine, which will evidently make anyplace in my head with a tear or leak light up, and then some kind of mesh being inserted and positioned over that lit-up area and secured in place. Then, after everything is sewn and patched, my intracranial pressure will be monitored to make sure there's enough of it, and not too much or too little. The whole process will require me to spend four or five days in the hospital. None of this seems like a good idea. But I'm not sure what else to do about this leak in my head, and shouldn't the doctors know better than I do how to fix it?

I'm waiting and waiting on a bed in the curtained-off room, hooked up to IVs in my hospital gown, and the ENT comes by from time to time, checking in. "Still leaking?" he asks, and I recognize this is supposed to be a joke. "Just checking!" he says, and continues, "You know, if you don't have a hole in your head before I go in, you'll definitely have one by the time I'm done. Think about it." He taps the protective guard rails on the bed and strolls out. I'm concerned. I talk to Gil. None of this seems okay. The next time the ENT strolls by, we ask what the hold-up is, why the wait, and he says it's almost time, and again introduces some doubt into the process, reminding me that this is my call. I don't like the feeling I'm getting, like this surgery is a thing I'm forcing him to do. It doesn't seem right, and I feel less confident that this is the right decision. He and Gil confer, and Gil says they're waiting for the room, but there's a chance I won't have the surgery today after all, that instead we'll just do the blood patch, the "voodoo" procedure the other doctor described. I keep waiting, and my vitals keep being monitored, and the crook of my arm aches where the IV lives now, and it's cold and I stare at the ceiling and can't sleep. Finally, after hours of waiting, the ENT comes back.

"I have bad news and bad news," he says. The bad news is, we are not going to do the through-the-face surgery. He just doesn't feel confident enough that that's where the leak is. And the other bad news is that we can't do the blood patch: The anesthesiology team isn't set up for it; they say they don't do them here in the hospital anyway, blood patches are done on an outpatient basis, in a clinic, which is in a different location. So after waiting all day, being hooked up to machines all day, after stressing all day over whether I'm making the right call, I'm free to go. The ENT says to call to set something up with the pain clinic where blood patches are done, but Gil isn't having it. Something needs to be set up *for* us, and it needs to happen now. The ENT strolls out and Gil goes after him, and I close my eyes as someone takes my IV out, removes the blood pressure cuff from my other arm. Eventually Gil returns, a resident comes in to take my information to facilitate an appointment with the pain clinic, and I go through my history all over again. My hospital records will somehow show this waste of a visit as my having had actual surgery, a fact that will have to be corrected every time I review my history with a new doctor.

8

I am back in bed, as I have been for weeks and weeks now, flat on my back, unable to read or watch TV or even have conversations, just kind of floating in this fog, trying hard to think.

I can't write—in my fog, I have that tipsy-drunk urge to chat, but also the tipsy-drunk cognitive impairment that makes typing almost impossible. Everything evaporates into the sensation of staring at the ceiling, because that's mostly what I do.

It's cruel, in a way, that I'm forced to have all this time and yet not be able to write. It's almost exactly my fantasy—for once, I'm free of the endless stuff that's never ever fully done: the chores and homework helping and school pickup and food preparation and dinner cleanup and laundry and housework and and and and—and yet I'm free from having to feel guilty, because I'm literally unable to do those things. It's seemingly the perfect scenario: I could write and not feel guilty about someone else picking up the slack of all the things that are left undone.

Yet I can't write, and no one's picking up the slack. My brain is too bruised from banging around in my skull without a cushion to do anything, and during those rare times when I'm forced to venture downstairs, I descend to find that no one else has done anything either. Everything is exactly as I left it weeks before, a tribute to the last time I'd been upright: the cat puke a hard crust on the floor, the dust fortified into corners, the dishes towering unscraped in the sink. I feel torn upon seeing this, some faraway, fog-padded part of me feeling humiliated, angry; and yet at the same time strangely energized, the ever-rationalizing part of my brain telling me *You can just clean everything up! What a great idea!* as I attempt to straighten up the mess, so happy to have a project, some measure of usefulness. Until the headache reasserts itself with a vengeance, reminding me that I can't trust my brain, that I shouldn't ever think that anything I think is a good idea, and I go back to bed, where I'm greeted by the strange neurological punishments of having been upright: the nauseous rush, the pressure on the left side of my head that's always followed by my arms disappearing and my words not speaking and my tears crying in too-loud sobs I can't control.

I can't write, but I can sometimes think, a little, about things I've written. Before this whole thing, I'd been working on a few projects. One was a novel set in the 1930s, during the Works Progress Administration era, about a pianist struggling to come into her own as an artist. Another was about a teen music prodigy who abandons her studies at a crucial point, runs away to meet up with a person she fell in love with on a video game server, tries to figure out who she is if she no longer does the thing she's done her whole life. And another was about a young woman, training as a pianist at a prestigious conservatory, suddenly sidelined by a mysterious illness doctors struggle to diagnose but which she fears she's brought on herself, fears she's using as a way to hide from the difficulties of her life, fears she's actually dying, fears she's pretending to be a person who's dying to escape having to be a person who's living.

The larger trend of these stories and how they relate to my current situation is not lost on me.

I'd most recently been working on revising the 1930s novel, the one about the woman whose artist husband had forbidden her to play, and how she found her way back to music after repression, depression, a suicide attempt, hospitalization. I'd had feedback that the story felt "too small," so I'd been working on trying to enlarge it. I changed the voice. I wrote a lot about time, the experience of time and how it changes when you're performing music, and how it changes when you're sick, when you're in the alternate universe of medications and bed rest, when you're in recovery, when you're once again part of the normal world.

In a way, this CSF leak of mine is almost research. Because here I am, outside of normal time. In the world outside my bedroom, life continues. Alarms go off in the mornings, the mail comes, dinner is made, appointments are kept. But in here, time is different. I feel closer to my main character than I ever had during the writing process as I lie in my bed, unable to think clearly or do anything that requires thinking and sitting up at the same time, like playing the piano, like writing, like parenting, like living my life.

There was a lot I'd gotten right about time, I'm discovering, the way I'd written about it for my protagonist. The way time moves when you're very sick, the way you can make days pass simply by closing your eyes, the way you float endlessly into the future, arriving from who knows how long ago in the past. The way time bores you but, due to your sickness, you don't mind being bored.

The way you can stare at the ceiling and not be impatient with the way absolutely nothing happens. The way music moves through time and how the sound exists in one moment, and then the next, and the next, and the next, and how we're able to fool ourselves into thinking it's a whole *thing*, when really it's just a stuttering passage, a succession of moments pretending to be seamless. Sickness is like that, making it easy to glide through time as if it's not perpetually one moment stitched to another, landing us foggily in the midst of the next moment until we realize, *Yes, of course, here I am.*

What I didn't get was the impotence. The way time makes you a prisoner. The way you must lie there knowing that mail is being delivered, that dinner needs to be made, that appointments need to be kept, and you cannot get it or make it or keep them. The way time heals you in real time, and you can't make it go faster. The way you're stuck, lying down, staring at the ceiling, feeling your way through the fog, waiting as one moment moves from the next to the next to the next.

Or the dependence, the way you must rely on favors from friends and strangers and the estranged. Your son's classmate's mother, whom you barely know, who volunteers to drive him home every day. Your daughter's friend's parents, who make food and bring it over in carefully labeled containers. The friend you haven't heard from in almost a year, who offers to take the kids, who orders in dinner. Your soon-to-be-ex-in-laws, who stay for a week when your soon-to-be-ex-husband can't, who straighten up what's been left a mess and cook things you normally wouldn't want to eat but devour now, lying on your side, since you can't sit up, with gratitude.

I try playing the piano once, during those staring-at-the-ceiling, time-bound, writing-less days when I rarely get out of bed, when I have maybe five, ten minutes of being upright before the pain sets in. I need to know if I'm still me. And so I go downstairs and sit down at the piano as a kind of test. I rush through thirty seconds of a Chopin nocturne, sketching it more than playing it. It feels like I'm listening to myself underwater, moving underwater, my brain moving so slowly, slower than my fingers, but I'm able to play it, I'm still me, and then my time is up, the pain returns, the pressure in my head unbearable.

9

May 2015

A week before my forty-fourth birthday, I have the "voodoo" procedure. I google it beforehand and find a PDF brochure titled "Let's Talk About Epidural Blood Patch Information" with a stock photo of a very sad-looking woman holding her head in her hands. As the neuro-ophthalmologist had told me, the epidural blood patch is similar to the kind of epidural administered in childbirth—only instead of a giant needle piercing your back with sweet pain relief, you're injected with your own blood, which they extract from you at roughly the same time you're being shishkabobbed in the back. The only plus side of this procedure versus the epidural I had during childbirth is that after this one, I do not also have to have a baby.

Arranging this is only slightly less stressful than my aborted surgical procedure. The day of the non-surgery, Gil and the ENT speak with the anesthesiology team about getting me set up at the pain center for a blood patch, and by the time we leave the hospital, everything is arranged, everything seems to be in place. Then the next day, just as I'm about to leave for my epidural blood patch appointment, I receive a call from the pain center: A team of doctors has reviewed my files and decided I don't need the procedure after all, have a good day. Gil calls them back, using his doctor powers to argue with them, and finally the head of the pain center agrees to see me—as long as I agree to take migraine medication over the weekend to see if it helps my headache. I'm irritated by this request, as I know it will be fruitless, but I take the medication as prescribed, and, predictably, feel nothing other than fatigue and the constant pain that is my life now.

Finally arriving at the pain center, no more calls to deter us, no more hoops to jump through, the head anesthesiologist welcomes us into his office, his exam table thoughtfully arranged for me as a flat bed. I climb on and apologize for having to talk to him while lying down, but it's all I can do. I'm weepy already from having been upright to get myself ready to come here, from walking from the car to the office building. Gil and the anesthesiologist talk above me as I lie on the exam table, saying words like *fluoroscopy* and *incidence* and *recovery rate*. They talk about my narrow escape from through-the-face-brain surgery, about how the migraine meds didn't make my headache go away, how my symptoms are "classic CSF leak," the positional aspect of the headache, the occipital pain. They both urge me to have this blood patch done. "I can do it today," the head anesthesiologist tells me, "or you can wait until Wednesday, when I'll have the room for fluoroscopy, it's up to you." I look at Gil, who tells me he thinks I should do it, and that I should do it today. I listen to them debate fluoroscopy versus no fluoroscopy, and eventually I realize they are waiting for me to say something. I'm crying, I don't know what to say. I'm terrified of this procedure and I don't want to have to do it. But it feels like it might be my only choice. "I don't know," I say, but Gil says, "You're in bad shape. I think you should do it. Like, as soon as possible. Today." And I can't argue with that.

I'm brought back to a curtained area, patient spaces separated by curtains on tracks, like in an ER. Not a lot of privacy, but then the place is basically empty this early on a Monday morning. I'm given a gown to change into, *leave it open in the back*, and I lie down on the gurney, watching people walk purposefully past the undrawn curtains around my bed. The anesthesiologist returns with a tray of alarming-looking needles and another person, a medical resident, he says, introducing her. I'm momentarily alarmed: "Shouldn't there be more people?" But no, he tells me. It's a two-person job. And so they sit me up, my entire head a ball of pain, and the resident straps a rubber tourniquet around my arm and asks me to make a fist as the anesthesiologist swabs my lower back with something cold, then needles it in several places with lidocaine. Soon, the resident is extracting blood from my arm, blood that must be used immediately, and I am made to lean forward as the anesthesiologist hunts for the right spot to stab me in the back with a giant needle and deliver that blood.

"I can feel that," I say at one point, as I lean on the resident's chest and fight off the go-toward-the-light tunnel vision brought on by having my blood drawn and my back skewered, and the excruciating headache brought on by sitting up. "Some pressure?" the doctor asks. "No, the needle," I say. "It's just pressure," he says. "It's the needle, I can feel it," I say. I start to pass out and they both yell questions at me to keep me awake. "How long have you lived here? What do you do? How many kids do you have? What did they do for you for Mother's Day?" My arms are tingling and my brain feels like it's getting smaller and smaller as I try to form words. *Seventeen years, I can't, I can't, write books, I can't, two, I can't, I can't, nothing, nothing, nothing, they didn't do anything I can't.*

"How old are your kids?" The doctor asks me, and the irony of it finally hits me, my worry about this illness making me a bad mother, being caused by being a bad mother, by being weak. *Dura mater* is the full name of the thing that tore in me. It means "tough mother."

They ask me to tell them when it's too much pressure, and I cry as I feel the needle jabbing some nerve and a heaviness in my back and finally yes, it's too much pressure, too much pressure in my back, too much pressure to be the one who has to decide how much pressure is too much pressure, to have it be my decision, my call, to have everything left up to me.

They lay me back onto the table and tell me I'm fine, that I did better than they'd expected (what had they expected?), and my headache is, for the moment, gone—but then it often subsides from lying down, so I can't be sure it's truly been banished. I'm foggy still, still unable to think like I used to be able to think, and exhausted from the blood pressure drop and the tears, and my back weeping what I hope isn't blood, though I can see the floor dotted with it, smears and drops they haven't bothered to clean up yet. I lie there on the cold table for an hour and then limp to the car to go home, my lower back and right leg a nerve map of pain. "You should be fine in a few days," the doctor says before I leave. "If you're not, we can do another one. Second blood patches have a success rate of over 95 percent." I tell him that I hope I never have to have another blood patch ever again, but he just shrugs and smiles and says, "Well, let me know. It's your call."

Days after the procedure I am out of bed, my back heavy, my right leg twinging, because the doctor has called and told me to be out of bed, as I can tolerate it, and because I have noticed that now when I lie down, my headache—oh yes, even after this procedure, I still have a headache—becomes intolerable. This is normal, the doctor tells me, it is normal for my head to feel like a blown-up balloon, to feel pressure behind my eyes and nose, to feel the genuinely unpleasant sensation of something like a deadly python squeezing my brain. This version of the headache is the Opposite-Day version of what I've been experiencing up until now: It used to be low, infiltrating the base of my skull; now it's high, in the front of my face. It used to improve a little when I lay flat; now lying flat makes me feel as though my head is about to explode. Caffeine used to make me feel better; now it makes the headache pain worse. "This happens sometimes," the doctor tells me over the phone. "Give it a few days to settle, give it time." I move slowly, but I move, and I try to stay upright instead of flat, and I try to drink less caffeine, and I try to give it time, because the doctor tells me this thing he's done is the thing that will fix me, so I must be fixed, right?

"How will I know if I need another patch? How will I know if this one doesn't work?" I ask him, and he says it's too early to tell. My head is now a balloon, ready to pop, and the headache is everywhere, and I am giving it time, but time seems to be colluding with the mystery of this thing to draw out the suspense. I wait for it all to settle as I grapple with the new contours of my pain, trying to ignore the dread that settles in instead that even though I am supposed to be fixed, I am not fixed, and perhaps not fixable.

10

All of us have a kind of primordial ocean in our heads, keeping our brains aloft on its current. This ocean of cerebrospinal fluid is generated continuously in the depths of our brains, produced by the choroid plexuses within the third and fourth ventricles. It suffuses and surrounds our brains, providing buoyancy, and bathes our spinal cords, lubricating the entirety of the central nervous system. Like the deep ocean, much of this has been nearly impossible to observe firsthand. The history of cerebrospinal fluid has been centuries of murky guesswork, increasingly deeper dives, usually by solo divers, revealing glimpses of an alien landscape, the dark waters of a humanoid ocean floor patrolled by impossible creatures, the hulls of failed ships transformed into coral reefs, nature reclaiming its space.

There is cerebrospinal fluid within us before we even technically have either a brain or a spine. It comes before thought, before mind, before brain, before even the development of those choroid plexuses in the ventricles of the brain that will eventually take over the process of circulating and generating this fluid, before any of us are recognizable as human. It exists in three-week-old embryos in the form of fluid within the neural tube that will eventually become the brain and central nervous system; by the fourth week, the first choroid plexus, a network of blood vessels and cells, develops in the fourth ventricle. Eventually this structure begins to produce and release cerebrospinal fluid continuously, as it will for the rest of our lives.

This isn't a thing that we can consciously control. Like the deep ocean, it is its own mystery. There are tides to cerebrospinal fluid production, peaks in its manufacture during the day and night to which none of us will ever likely be sensitive, unless something, mysteriously, goes wrong. Like the deep ocean, it used to be thought that this water in our brains was just water, and not something teeming with life, with its own purpose. And yet, like the deep ocean, it has also been the subject of myths and legends, with speculation about its mystical properties, assertions that this magical fluid might actually be the river of life, the source of consciousness, the place where the soul resides. We understand more now about the anatomy and structure and purpose of the brain and central nervous system; we have a more fleshed-out understanding than we did in the days where notions of these things were like maritime maps with drawings of dragons and mermaids and other fantastical creatures to mark spots of danger and obscurity. But in some ways the reality of what lies in its depths is stranger than anything we imagined; like the ocean, no dragons or mermaids, but instead merely the weirdness of furry-clawed crabs living 5,000 feet deep in hydrothermal vents, blind lobsters, light-producing deep-sea anglerfish, giant squid, bioluminescent octopi, isopod crustaceans, and other creatures that have been inhabiting this world, unbeknownst to us, for longer than humans have existed. It's only recently that we have learned there's more to cerebrospinal fluid than just providing a cushion to our brains, allowing them to float, acting as a link to our distant, primeval beginnings of life in the sea billions of years ago.

The earliest documentation of cranial cerebrospinal fluid was discovered on a papyrus fragment found in 1862 by the Egyptologist Edwin Smith. When the papyrus was finally translated in the 1930s, it revealed a medical history written by the Egyptian physician Imhotep around 3000 BC, detailing an account of a patient with open head trauma. According to Imhotep's report, the patient's skull fracture and meningeal rupture "[broke] open his fluid in the interior of his head."

Other ancient physicians observed this brain fluid but did not always agree about its purpose—or even its existence. While Hippocrates (460–375 BC) described "water" surrounding the brain, the anatomist Galen (AD 130–200) noted the presence of "excremental liquid" in the ventricles of the brain, but dismissed it, believing those cavities to primarily contain not fluid but a gas-like *spiritus animalis* that provided energy throughout the body and was the key to human consciousness.

Andreas Vesalius, a sixteenth-century anatomist from the Netherlands considered the founder of modern human anatomy, described the cerebral ventricles and choroid plexus, and noted the presence of "brain water," estimating that its volume was as much as one-sixth the volume of the brain. (Modern MRI studies have revealed that cerebrospinal fluid accounts for 18 percent of total brain volume.) He also, strikingly, broke with the Aristotelian tradition of believing the heart to be the center of the soul, and the source of feelings and emotions in the body: He posited that the brain and nervous system was where the mind was, and was the originator of emotion, and made the bold claim that nerves originate from the brain, and not the heart. (He also put to rest the medical belief put forth by Galen that women have fewer teeth than men.)

The Venetian physician Nicolò Massa noted in his 1536 publication *Anatomiae Libri Introductorius* that there appeared to be fluid within cerebral ventricles. More than one hundred years later, Humphrey Ridley published the first English-language manuscript about brain anatomy, which also made note of the presence of cerebrospinal fluid within the ventricles. The anatomist Antonio Maria Valsalva, whose name we know from his eponymous maneuver, and whose primary interest was the workings of the human ear, in 1692 described cerebrospinal fluid as existing within the subarachnoid space around the spinal cord.

In Italy in the 1700s, Domenico Cotugno literally turned on its head the then-traditional method of performing autopsies (severing the head from the rest of the body before dissecting the brain), by instead keeping the bodies intact and positioning them upside down. This allowed him to observe fluid beneath the dura mater, the tough covering surrounding the brain and spinal cord, and within the ventricles of the brain. For a time, due to his discovery, cerebrospinal fluid was called "liquor Cotunnii," or Cotugno's liquid. Still, it wasn't until 1842 that the French physician François Magendie coined the term "cerebrospinal fluid" and discovered a means of measuring its pressure, laying the foundation for the development of cerebrospinal fluid dynamic research. And yet even then Magendie's contemporaries, including neurologists Albert von Haller and Moritz Romberg, argued that the brain's networked series of cavities—the ventricles—were filled with some kind of humid gas instead of fluid.

Working in isolation, somewhat outside of the medical profession, was a Swedish engineer turned anatomist turned theologian named Emanuel Swedenborg, who between 1741 and 1744 came up with a visionary description of cerebrospinal fluid that wasn't widely recognized until his work on the subject was published posthumously in 1887. His insights into cerebrospinal fluid and the cerebral cortex coincided with a time in his life when he experienced a spiritual awakening that led him to believe he had been appointed by Jesus Christ to reform Christianity, starting a religious movement that continues to this day. Somehow, along the way, he managed to investigate the mysteries of CSF, referring to it as "spiritous lymph" and "highly gifted juice." In a kind of fluid-filled echo of the ancient conclusions Galen held about the gaseous animal spirits of human consciousness residing in the pockets of the brain, Swedenborg believed the cerebrospinal fluid to be where the soul resides. Swedenborg also greatly influenced Andrew Taylor Still, the founder of osteopathy (a branch of medicine concerned with managing health through the manipulation of bones, joints, and muscles). Both Still and Swedenborg believed in the idea of cerebrospinal fluid as the location of the soul, and vital to overall health. As Still put it: "The cerebrospinal fluid is the highest known element in the human body. He who is able to reason will see that this great river of life must be tapped and the withering field irrigated at once or the harvest of health is forever lost." Other osteopaths, such as Randolph Stone, who went on to found something he called polarity therapy—a kind of holistic energy healing practice—also characterized CSF as a spiritual "liquid medium for . . . life energy radiation, expansion, and contraction." Stone said, "Where this is present, there is life and healing with normal function. Where this primary and essential life force is not acting in the body, there is obstruction, spasm, or stagnation and pain, like gears which clash instead of meshing in their operation." Even modern-day naturopaths such as New Mexico doctor Robert Stevens subscribe to this view of cerebrospinal fluid as something spiritual and holy: "On the physical level, cerebrospinal fluid becomes the physical carrier of the wisdom of the Soul. This fluid conveys the sound and light energies of the Soul throughout the physical body. CSF expresses this highest vibratory rate and intelligence to the whole physical body."

Outside of the community of visionaries and spiritual osteopaths, for hundreds of years the consensus was, among most physicians, that the primary function of cerebrospinal fluid was to protect and cushion the brain. It took until the early twentieth century for cerebrospinal fluid to be recognized as playing a crucial role in the function of the entire central nervous system. Harvey Cushing, the father of neurosurgery, called this the "third circulation" in a 1925 paper that established CSF physiology as a crucial aspect of neuroscience. He saw the flow of cerebrospinal fluid as a circulatory system similar to vascular and lymphatic circulation, and introduced the idea of cerebrospinal fluid and its circulation as a kind of lymphatic system for the brain, clearing out waste. He suggested that cerebrospinal fluid flows through the ventricles, cisterns, and subarachnoid space, and is reabsorbed into the blood at the arachnoid villi—from *arachne*, meaning spider, and *villus*, shaggy hair, these are spidery, hair-like projections of fibrous tissue protruding from the arachnoid membrane.

There are three membranes surrounding the brain and spinal cord, collectively known as the meninges, and the dura mater is the outermost of the three. These membranes—the pia mater (*tender mother*, attached to the surface of the brain and spinal cord), the arachnoid mater (*spider-like mother*, the middle layer, named for its spiderweb appearance), and the dura mater (*tough mother*, named for its durability and strength)—protect the central nervous system. The dura is, true to its name, normally a quite dense and fibrous connective tissue, which functions somewhat like a sac encapsulating the brain and spinal cord, extending to the sacrum, beyond the base of the spinal cord.

It's the dura that keeps the cerebrospinal fluid contained. The fluid moves within it, pulsing from the inner recesses of the brain, and traveling along the length of the spinal cord, coating the entire central nervous system. When the dura mater is pierced or torn from trauma or injury or medical procedures gone wrong, cerebrospinal fluid can seep out, reducing the pressure of the rest of the fluid around the brain. Often the only sign that this has happened is a headache that becomes worse when sitting or standing, as being upright reduces the pressure around the brain even more. Women in labor who receive epidural anesthesia, where a needle is used to inject anesthetic into the space just outside the dura, can experience this if the anesthesiologist pushes the needle just slightly too far, piercing the dura. People requiring spinal injections, where a needle is deliberately inserted through the dura to deliver anesthetic, or lumbar punctures are also at risk. Often these small holes, made by very fine needles, repair themselves or otherwise seal over and resolve over days or weeks; when they do not, intervention is required. Instances like these, where the site of the leak is known, are more straightforward to address; spontaneous cerebrospinal fluid leaks—those not caused by deliberate or accidental needle puncture—are harder to track down, more difficult to source, and thus trickier to repair.

The first case of post-lumbar puncture headache was noted in the nineteenth century. In the early part of the twentieth century, doctors began documenting cases involving patients suffering from symptoms resembling that of a post-puncture headache, but without the puncture. These low CSF volume headaches came to be known as spontaneous intracranial hypotension, or spontaneous spinal CSF leaks. The condition became more recognized throughout the latter half of the twentieth century through pioneering work by neurologists like the late Bahram Mokri, who spent much of his forty years at the Mayo Clinic researching and treating cerebrospinal fluid leaks; but even today a solid body of research on the subject is only just beginning to emerge. This makes it an exciting time for researchers, as nearly any new data about spinal CSF leaks breaks new ground, medically speaking; and a frustrating time for clinicians, as there is little in the way of hard facts to offer patients in terms of prognosis and recovery. The team of doctors at Cedars-Sinai in Los Angeles, including neurosurgeon Wouter I. Schievink, and the team of doctors at Duke University, including neuroradiologists Linda Gray-Leithe and Peter Kranz, are the current top clinician-researchers in the field, pushing for and performing valuable research, inventing and refining pioneering treatments, mentoring other physicians in the diagnosis and management of cerebrospinal fluid leaks, and learning from the patients they treat.

The history of evolving medical knowledge of cerebrospinal fluid—its importance, its function, the problems that emerge when the system it's a part of becomes compromised or otherwise out of balance—is one of independent discoveries, sometimes the same discoveries made by different people at different times in different parts of the world. Even now, the challenge is to disseminate basic facts and protocols for treatment among doctors of different specialties, so that this obscure body of knowledge can be more widely shared, and offer patients better avenues toward treatment. It is somewhat telling that the first major symposium on spontaneous intracranial hypotension to take place anywhere in the world, bringing together researchers, neurologists, primary care doctors, nurses, physical therapists, other medical professionals, and patients, happened only as recently as October 2017.

The great sea within us, whose tides peak in the mid-to-late afternoon and in the early hours of the morning, which ebbs and flows according to its own mysterious process, is a secret, pooling in and around our brains. "The soul swims in the CSF," the naturopaths say, and perhaps there is some truth to it. Certainly there is some complex function this fluid serves, some purpose it has that we notice only in those moments when it affects us adversely, swelling our heads at permanent high tide, or draining away through a tear too small for even a mechanical eye to see. And the work keeps going, physicians diagnosing, specialists scanning, patients describing, all of us swimming toward understanding.

11

May 2015

B ack at the hospital, I know where to go now. I know where all the couches are where a person can lie down because her brain fluid is leaking; the place in the waiting area with the double-wide chairs, wide enough to wedge yourself in sideways, your head resting on the wooden arms; the not-too-conspicuous spot with a cushioned bench that's not too impolite to sprawl out on. But today, two weeks after the blood patch, I am okay. I don't need to lie down. I'm able to walk to the check-in kiosk and smile, give my name, sit down in a regular-wide chair, listen to the sounds of the talk show on the television behind me, hear an old couple to my left argue about going to jury duty, the woman scolding the man for not getting a doctor's note, telling him he'd be arrested for not showing up. It's not at all like the last time I was here. This time, I answer questions. I don't struggle to sit upright, to walk. I smile and make small talk and understand what people say to me.

This time, I'm here to have another CT scan and films because of that pesky dens fracture the doctors noticed in my second cervical vertebra. Normally, they said, this is the kind of thing they see in car accidents or terrible trauma, and normally it's the kind of thing they see acutely. In other words, it's not the kind of thing you normally just walk around with. It appears to be a very old fracture, but the question is whether or not it has any involvement in what's been going on, whether it has anything to do with the leak or the pain in my head. I can't imagine that it does; I've ridden roller coasters and done headstands in yoga for years without any consequences. Unless this CSF leak *is* the consequence, finally catching up with me after so many years of recklessness.

I know what this old fracture is from: My sisters and I fooling around, doing gymnastics in the family room when I was seven, eight. There was a piece of furniture there that had come with the house, a wooden bar stand, just taller than a tall dresser, and we liked to use it to play house, setting up our dolls and animals on the shelves inside it. One day, reenacting the gymnastics moves we'd learned in class, we dared each other to try more and more risky things. I was brave then, or braver than I am now, and so I stood on top of that bar, my hands reaching up to graze the low ceiling, and volunteered to do a flip off it onto the floor. Never mind that I'd never once in my life done a flip. There was a thin gym mat there for me to land on, I could do it. My sisters looked skeptical, but that only fueled my confidence.

I remember the leap, the free-fall feeling of wishing I could take back my boasting, my stupid bravado, the expressions on my sisters' faces as I jumped off.

I landed on the back of my head. I hadn't flipped enough in the air to get all the way around. And I had the wind knocked out of me a little bit. But the main priority was that we not get in trouble, so even though I cried, and even though it hurt, we agreed not to say anything to our parents. Later I told my mom I'd somehow tripped walking up the steps to the laundry room and hit my head. I think she gave me aspirin. I think I went to bed early. My sisters and I never talked about it again. A few times in my life I've thought about that moment, how lucky I was. One slight shift of gravity and I could have died. I could have literally broken my neck. Instead, evidently, I just fractured it.

I have the X-rays done first. Once I'm gowned, I'm made to stand against a metal square, with a smaller metal square in front of me, a light shining into my eyes. They have me look straight ahead, chin slightly up; then with my mouth so wide open it feels like my jaw might get stuck; then facing to the side with my head normal, then down, then tilted back. After that I'm escorted to the CT/MRI scan area. The last time I'd been there, for an MRI, I'd curled in a chair, trying my best to get horizontal, crying from the pain. Today I sit with the other gowned patients in the waiting area, CNN on the overhead TV, the women who need contrast for their procedures commiserating over the terrible drink they're required to ingest. Mocha, berry, banana—all, apparently, equally awful. A woman my age is given two bottles of the stuff by a tech. "Both of these?" she asks, apprehension clear on her face. "Yep," he tells her, "but it's okay, you have forty-five minutes to get them down." She winces open the first one and puts a straw in, and the other women sad-smile in solidarity.

I've been having a kind of sharp, stabbing pain on the side of my head, just behind my right ear, all morning. I google "sharp stabbing pain" and learn that "ice-pick headaches" are a thing. I feel myself panicking a little: *Is my head hurting like it used to?*

I've been upright since 7 A.M., that's a long time, is the leak back? Can a person die from ice-pick headaches? Are ice-pick headaches a sign of a brain tumor? Are ice-pick headaches a sign of a failed epidural blood patch? I reminded myself not to google "failed epidural blood patch." I've done it before. The discussion boards are terrifying. I try some deep breathing and tell myself it's normal to feel anxious, especially since the last time I was here I was in so much pain, but that I'm okay now, and even if I'm not, guess what, I'm in a hospital, so, yes: Everything will be okay, one way or another.

Eventually it's my turn. I'm brought back to the room and placed on a movable slab, my head resting in a cradle extension sticking off the end of the table. A nurse tells me not to move or swallow, and then remarks that hearing that probably makes me want to move or swallow. And even though I hadn't wanted to move or swallow before she said that, I suddenly feel the urge. "You can swallow when the table is still," the nurse says, "so just try to save it for when the table isn't moving." I try to move and swallow extra before the scan starts to get it out of my system. With my eyes closed tight against the light panic of being in a somewhat enclosed space, it's hard to tell when the table is moving or not. I swallow at one point, unable to hold off any longer, hoping the table stays still while I do it. Then it's all done, and I'm able to move freely and swallow whenever I want and change out of my gown and into my clothes and go back out into the world.

The last time I was here, I'd gone to the second floor landing, which always seemed to be more or less empty, and had lain on the couch for half an hour or so until I could face the five or ten minutes of being upright to hail a cab. Today I go to the food place in the lobby, get a snack, walk to the taxi stand like a normal person, and go home.

I feel so normal, but of course I'm not back to normal; my brain just thinks I am. And compared to even a week before, it's not wrong. Still, once home, I have to rest. I lie in bed, listening to a podcast, eventually falling asleep, the long chain of events of the French revolution narrating my dreams.

When I wake up, I decide to move. I've been "deconditioned," the doctors say, from so long in bed, and it's important for me to get up and walk around when I can, it's important for me to move. Last week, I walked around the house, cleaning, doing laundry, picking up. This week, I walk outside for five minutes, ten minutes, almost a mile. Once, as I returned home from one of these slow walks, I passed a woman trying to argue with a cranky toddler desperate to escape the stroller. "No! You must learn *patience*," the woman said, and I smirked, thinking, *Good luck with that, she's just a baby, you'll be saying that for years before she's actually capable of being patient*. But then as I continued slowly past them it hit me that sometimes you need to hear good advice for years and years before you are actually ready to take it. I'm healing slowly. I too must learn patience.

I end up walking two miles. I walk on the crowded streets, among people even, even though I have to go so slowly now. I browse in a clothing store, find two T-shirts for Nate—he's growing, I've noticed his clothes tight on him when he comes to my bed to hug me goodnight—and a dress for me maybe, and then ultimately decide not to buy anything at all. It's more like a dress rehearsal for actual shopping, for the patience of actual shopping. I'm going through the motions, I'm moving. It's important for me to move. And so I return home, listening to another podcast, trying to gauge the dull ache in the back of my head, my neck, to see how it's doing, thinking how strange it is to be walking around listening to a podcast instead of lying in bed listening to a podcast, unable to think clearly enough to do more than lie down and listen and let the voices keep me company.

12

My tentative experiments in normalcy have me hopeful for the first time since everything began. The brain-squeezing pressure that I had after the blood patch has begun to subside, and even though the more that front-top headache recedes, the more the familiar back-of-skull headache resurges—even though I still feel foggy and in more pain as the day goes on, even though I still need to rest—all of this feels like some kind of progress, some kind of change, which feels better than the purgatory of being suspended in time, in bed, waiting out the pain.

One afternoon I find myself at the piano, rifling through a book of Rachmaninoff preludes until I find one that seems familiar. From the looks of it, I must have tried to learn it a million years ago: The score has my fingerings and dynamics markings on every page, but

I don't remember ever performing it. It was probably something I'd attempted on my own, for fun, after the conservatory, unmoored without my old teacher, who likely never would have encouraged me to study it, with my small hands.

I decide to sight-read it. It's beautiful, in that way of Rachmaninoff preludes, but it's the kind of piece that's a struggle the entire way through, a melody with inner voices against a triplet accompaniment, a struggle against time. You have to fight with it to make it sound smooth and not plodding, or at least to make it not sound like you're playing two against three the whole time, which of course you are. You have to make it delicate and balanced, despite the wide jumps in the left hand that make it hard to control the tone, the inner voices in the right hand that sometimes carry the melody and other times are more a part of the left hand's story.

In a way, its beauty comes precisely from this struggle. This difficulty is the entire point of the piece, and to really play it, you can't ignore that difficulty. You can't make it smooth by glibly smoothing it over. Or, you can; but then the point is missed, then it's just a melody that's pretty and flows past you and then is gone. To really play it, to really understand it and make someone else understand it, you have to embrace the struggle of it.

Lots of pieces are a struggle for me, because of my too-small hands, and, after decades away from the kind of training I used to do, because of my rusty technique, my out-of-practice-ness, and no-longer-refined ears. And now of course because of this leak. But I try to remind myself to go as slowly as I need to, to keep the sound layers straight, to keep this part in front and that part behind, to remember where that jump starts and where this arpeggio lands, and so I go slowly and try to let the struggle be a struggle, to let myself be patient with it.

As the sound fills the room, I hear the buzz of the window whenever I hit a certain G, the cats jumping from the counter, the kids down the street playing ball outside. I keep making mistakes, but I try to be okay with that, to be patient with it, because that's the struggle, and because I'm reading music, I'm sitting up, I'm playing. And then I arrive at my favorite part, about halfway through, the part with these heartbreaking open sixths in the right hand, its mysterious, somber melody, and it surprises me when I get there, I'd let it sneak up on me, and I find myself weeping as I realize, *I'm sitting up, I'm playing, and my head doesn't hurt, and my arms are moving, and my fingers are moving, and I'm thinking, and my brain feels less foggy, and I can do this, I can still do this, I am doing this,* and the weeks and weeks of not being able to do anything finally reveal themselves to me as a hiding place for a giant repository of fear. To be able to play the piano like this—to be able to sit for more than a few minutes with my head only hurting a little, to be able to think and concentrate and process and react—even a month ago, that was impossible. And realizing at that moment that it is not only possible, it is actually happening, makes me overcome, overwhelmed. I cry all the way through the rest of the piece, through my mistakes and sloppy pedaling, through my clumsy articulation, all the way through to the end, to that moment of *Yes, of course, here I am,* where I let the sound of the last chord linger as my breath catches and I sob and sob and sob.

That novel I'd been working on for so long, that stupid endless story I couldn't get quite right, about the woman whose husband forbids her to play, her struggle to become well, to return to herself, to find the hidden music again—I'd written and rewritten countless times the scene where she finally finds a piano, where she confronts her new limitations at the instrument, where she tries to reconnect with herself and with the way she thinks, with who she is when she plays music. So many times I wrote it and revised it and reworked it and rethought it—*and I never got to this moment.* I wrote about her frustrations, her disappointments, her emotions upon being able to play again. But never that moment of hope. Of relief. Of realizing that she wasn't broken. Of realizing maybe she was going to be okay.

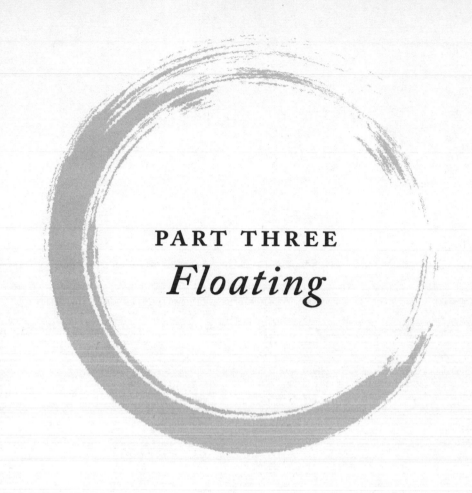

PART THREE
Floating

The hallmark manifestation of SIH [spontaneous intracranial hypotension] is positional headache . . . . And yet, there are many facets of the disease that are not straightforward and remain poorly understood. Underdiagnosis remains a major problem. Many physicians still are unaware of the disease, or have little to no experience in its management. This problem is compounded by the fact that variant clinical presentations exist . . . . Spinal CSF leaks, the presumed etiology in most cases, are never detected in some patients with clear manifestations of SIH, despite exhaustive investigation. Finally, treatment remains challenging. Many patients recover well from the disease, but substantial numbers of patients suffer relapses and may have to undergo multiple treatments . . . . For some, the consequences of these deficiencies in our understanding of SIH can be severe. Long-term disability, with the attendant emotional and economic consequences, can have life-altering effects for some sufferers of the disease.

—P.G. Kranz, L. Gray, and J.N. Taylor,
"CT-Guided Epidural Blood Patching of Directly
Observed or Potential Leak Sites for the Targeted
Treatment of Spontaneous Intracranial Hypotension,"
American Journal of Neuroradiology, May 2011

13

June 2015

Weeks after the blood patch, the cautious optimism I'd been feeling has begun to drain away, like the slow seep of cerebrospinal fluid leaking out of a spine. All the old symptoms are back, with only one slight change. The fog and the scraping, prickling feeling in my head; that's the same. The back-of-skull headache, though: That's on the left side now.

It's becoming clear to me that the blood patch has failed. I say "failed," that the blood patch has failed, that perhaps I have failed, because that is the terminology, I've come to learn, when the blood patch doesn't work. *Failure.* And yet the doctors I've seen haven't been able to accurately describe success.

"Voodoo," the neuro-ophth had called the blood patch, and when I'd asked why, he'd said, "Well, we don't really know how or why it works. Some people theorize it's something where the blood gets injected and then clots, and then basically that clump of blood floats up to where the leak is and just plugs up the hole." The anesthesiologist who performed the procedure had described it more as pinching the bottom of a balloon to hold it shut and prevent the air from escaping. "So, *not* tying the bottom of a balloon to keep the air in, but just *pinching* it shut, which could allow air to leak out still," I'd said, and he'd said "Yes, more or less."

I'm assuming that's what's happened, that the clump of blood didn't float up to where it should have, which seems unlikely anyhow; that the clump of blood didn't pinch shut the balloon of my spine hard enough to keep things from escaping. That this leak is still leaking, slower perhaps than before. The blood patch has failed, but as the familiar pain returns, it feels more like the failure is mine.

I meet with yet another neurosurgeon, this time to talk about whether or not the old fracture in my neck could have played any role in causing the CSF leak, or with my continuing symptoms. I am back to being limited to twenty minutes of upright time, twenty minutes of normalcy, before the headache pain returns, trenchant and sickly familiar. I'm weepy in the waiting area from sitting up too long, and once the nurse practitioner calls me in, I cry while telling her my history, telling her about the leak and how I'm worried it's back, that it never actually went away, that I don't want to have to endure the barbarism of another useless procedure, a voodoo curse, a blind injection, a waste of time that makes my head a balloon that can't float away.

The doctor comes in and performs the basic chitchat, the basic neurological exam. He shows me a model of the cervical spine, explaining what the normal anatomy looks like, and pointing out the difference between those normal things and what is happening in my actual, non-normal neck. He's reviewed my scans, and it appears I have a fracture in a growth plate that appears to be pretty old, lining up with my story of landing on my head when I was eight. He also says I have a thing where a bone that's supposed to be held in place by a ligament is actually fused to some other bone. Most likely I was born with it.

The basic point, though, is that since I'm not having pain in my arms or hands, or weakness, or any other symptoms other than this pain and brain fog due to the CSF leak, he doesn't think it's worth the risk of surgery to go in and fix either of those things. Especially since the surgery would leave me with a very limited range of motion. In fact, he doesn't think this stuff has anything to do with the leak. He says my vertebra dentata isn't toothy enough to have bitten through the dura, that while my weird neck situation could theoretically compress a nerve and cause occipital pain, similar to the low back-of-skull pain I have with this leak, my symptoms are more in line with a CSF leak than nerve compression. He says that a shot of pain-relief medicine called an occipital block could possibly help with my pain levels—but only if my occipital pain is actually due to this issue with my neck and not due to the low-pressure headache of a leak. Neither of us think this is a viable option for me, as it seems clear my pain is from the CSF leak and not from my strange neck situation, which was a secret only revealed in the hunt for the cause of this leak. He doesn't have any advice about the leak, or even any experience with CSF leaks, and suggests I follow up with some headache neurologist out in the suburbs who also doesn't have any experience with CSF leaks, so I thank him and smile politely but I understand that this is a dead end.

He'd laughed when I told him the story of my failed flip, how I stuck the landing right on the back of my head, how the first thing I said after I stopped crying was "We can't tell mom," how I didn't go to the doctor, just got some aspirin and went to bed. He'd said nowadays people are so jumpy they even take their pets to the ER, but back in the day you just did whatever and it was no big deal. Third-degree burn? Put some butter on it. I was lucky; I could have died. We were all lucky back then.

There's a CSF leak expert at Cedars-Sinai in Los Angeles. I found him through googling things about CSF leaks, things that usually led me to links for either abstracts of worst-case-scenario medical papers or sobering bulletin-board tales of years-long suffering posted by people who call themselves "leakers." There was a Q&A with this expert on one of these sites, and his name came up a few other times in my searches, usually in the context of being the doctor of last resort, the doctor who finally put all the pieces together and, sometimes, even fixed the problem. I am tempted to try to meet with him. I don't know whether my leak is leaky enough, if my case is bad enough to merit a last-resort doctor, if I am suffering enough to call myself a leaker. But if this leak really is still leaking, I need one person to oversee all this and figure out what's going on, rather than going from doctor to doctor to doctor, each with their own small piece of the puzzle that doesn't make sense in isolation.

Maybe I'm not still leaking, maybe the dull pain on my left side that feels just like the leak pain on my right side is a random thing, maybe I just didn't want hard enough for this blood patch to work, maybe I didn't hope hard enough or rest hard enough or not rest hard enough, maybe the stupid fortune-cookie fortune I got a few weeks ago was right when it said, "Enthusiasm can change the current situation." A part of my brain rejects that, floating up a thought that says *Fuck that fortune-cookie fortune*, but who knows if I can trust anything my brain tells me right now. I can't trust myself to make decisions. And yet I have to as the doctors shrug, as the neurosurgeon says my guess is as good as his, as Gil comes to my room to ask what to do about the kids, dinner, the messy house. *Your call. You decide. Up to you.*

14

This is not the first time I have been a difficult patient.

It is early fall 1990 and I am nineteen years old. I am sick, and no one knows what's wrong with me.

The gown gapes at my back, the crinkly examination table paper chills my bare thighs, my sockless feet swing in the silence. The rheumatologist paces a little as he thumbs through my file, and I stare out the window, wishing I could be outside, away, anywhere but here.

Everything is green here. The bus ride from Boston was a journey from gray and brown and brick-red to the dense green of trees forested together, the sun-polished green of well-kept lawns, the shifting green of leaves slowly being invaded by fall: the color of the suburbs. Arriving, I found the office tucked away like a witch's house in a fairy tale, shaded by thick, tall trees, marked by ivied walkways, a moat of luxuriously bright flowerbeds offering a ring of protection.

The thin paper crackles as I shift my weight, and the rheumatologist looks over his glasses at me.

"Why don't you get dressed now, and we'll chat in the other room when you're ready," he says. He's old and soft-spoken. He must be somebody's grandfather. His hands when he examined me were so gentle, yet firm; careful. The thought of that kindness makes my eyes sting as I put my clothes back on.

The other room isn't like a doctor's office at all. It's more like a room in somebody's fancy house, like a library, with low leather chairs, floor-to-ceiling bookshelves filled with burgundy and deep-green leather-bound books, dark wood grain everywhere I look, grand windows like in my piano teacher's studio. He sits behind a large desk, my file open in front of him, and smiles at me as I enter, waving me toward the chair.

"So, your pain level, on a scale of one to ten, is?"

This is a hard question to answer.

"Six or seven, I guess. Most days. It depends."

He nods.

"And the fatigue—does it interfere with your daily life?"

An easier question.

"Yes."

"And this started . . ."

"Well, the pain part started three months ago."

I could tell him exactly when. *June 28, 1990, 3:27 P.M.* I could tell him exactly how it started, how I felt it in my fingers first— not like the kind of fatigue that comes naturally after practicing piano for three hours, but actual pain, aches in all the bones of my fingers—then my wrists, then my arms. How it slowly moved to encompass my whole body, like I was being swallowed, hands first, by a snake. How it hasn't stopped hurting ever since.

What I can't tell him is why.

He nods again, leans back in his chair, holding the details of my life in his hands. The file should be thicker, I think. But then again, I haven't been allowed to read it; maybe it says everything it needs to.

"Cognitive issues? Fuzzy thinking, problems coming up with the right words, that sort of thing? Memory problems?"

"Yes," I say. "Like I'm thinking underwater. If that makes any sense." Words swim away from me all the time. I am heavy with gravity.

"You're a music student?"

A deceptively easy question. But this way lies the trap.

"Yes. Piano."

"Ah, New England Conservatory?" He smiles.

"No, the Boston Conservatory." He frowns. Perhaps he doubts me. More likely he's never heard of it. "New England Conservatory is our deadly rival."

I'm joking, but his eyebrows raise.

"Quite a high-pressure field, classical music. Competitive?"

This is the trick question, even though he has cleverly disguised it as something else.

Already I feel the anxiety rising. Already I want to head him off at the pass, tell him not to assume that I'm sick because I'm stressed or under pressure, not to assume I'm the kind of person who complains about pain, who simply gets tired, who lets being tired ruin her life, who wastes doctors' time with petty complaints about being tired and in pain when really she could just work harder. But I can't say any of that, because then I'll not only confirm to him that I am stressed and under pressure, I'll confirm to him that I am high-strung and neurotic, and then I'll be sick because I'm just a sick person, and he'll give me the same "You're a teenager, you're a musician, you're just a girl, just try to relax" conversation I've had with a million other doctors and shoo me out the door, and I'll still be in pain—in so much pain—and still I won't know why, and still we will dance around the unspoken question I know he really wants to ask, the question I ask myself all the time, the question everyone dances around but never actually comes out and says, which is: *Are you crazy?*

But he surprises me by not bothering to wait for an answer.

"Do you have friends at school?" he asks.

This is a suspicious question. If I say yes, that will mean I am normal. If I tell the truth and say not really, I will not be normal, even though at the conservatory it is normal to not really have friends, because we are all too busy practicing, and because we are all in competition with one another. If I am normal, that factors into the diagnostic equation, becomes a question mark, in fact: How could a normal person be sick with such mysterious symptoms? If I am not normal, that itself becomes a symptom. Perhaps even a cause.

"Yes," I say. "I have friends."

I'm not technically lying.

"Do you have a boyfriend?"

This is the most difficult question. I don't even know how to begin to answer it. How would he answer it, if he were here?

"Kind of?"

My right shin throbs, my left arm, too, in concert. My hands ache, but not the practicing kind of ache: The pain ache. I feel it in the top of my left wrist, just beneath my right thumb, the knuckles of both hands. I'm so tired.

He smiles. "It's not a trick question. Either you have a boyfriend or you don't."

His friendliness about it makes me feel for a moment as though we are not doctor and patient, but just amicable strangers making the kind of small talk you have to make at parties or holiday dinners when you are old enough to be out in the world but not yet old enough to be taken seriously.

"Are you sexually active?" he asks.

A humiliating question. This isn't small talk, I remind myself, no matter how much it feels like I'm sitting in somebody's grandfather's study. These are doctorly questions. I have to be vigilant.

"No."

This is the truth. But he doesn't even look up at me, just jots something down in my file.

"Well, then that answers my previous question: No boyfriend," he says. "Have you ever been in the past?"

"Excuse me?" I ask.

"Sexually active."

"Oh." The most humiliating question. "No."

He closes my file folder, lays it on the desk. Taps his pen a few times as he looks around the room. My bones ache. I hope I'll be able to sleep on the bus ride back. Finally he looks at me.

"Well. I have a few recommendations to make. For one thing, I'd like to have some further blood work done." He looks through the file for just a moment. "I'll give your doctor a call and go over my thoughts with her, and then we can get you scheduled for another blood draw. It's just a hunch, but I think I might have an inkling about what's going on with you. The blood panel will let us know if I'm on the right track."

"You mean." My mouth is dry suddenly, and the words are so thick, a milkshake I can barely coax through a straw. "You might have a diagnosis?"

He waves his hand, a conductor tamping forte down to mezzo forte.

"I wouldn't go that far. In the meantime, we can start with better pain management." He scribbles something on a prescription pad, tears off the paper, and hands it to me. "This may help, though it might also make you drowsy, so you might want to try taking it in the evening at first, so you can see how you tolerate it."

The paper is filled with hieroglyphs, squiggles and lines I can't decipher. *This could help me*, I think, and the realization strangles my heart for a moment. I haven't allowed myself to think of how much I want to be helped. My leg flares with pain again and I fold the prescription paper in half and put it in my music bag and try not to let myself be flooded with hope.

"Do you have any questions?" he asks.

This is the trickiest of trick questions.

If I ask too many questions—even if I ask just one too-probing question—I risk being seen as "difficult." One of "those" patients. If I don't ask any questions at all, I risk being seen as unmotivated, uncaring, affectless. All of it goes into the file, becomes another piece of the story of why I am sick.

But I am buoyed by the paper he just handed to me, comforted by the way he looks, sitting there in his comfortable chair, in this doctor's office unlike any doctor's office I've been in in the past few months, his glasses sliding down his nose as he watches me with concern just like a doctor in a Norman Rockwell painting.

"Yes, actually," I say, summoning my voice. "One question, really."

"Of course," he says.

"If the medicine. This medicine you've prescribed me."

I take a deep breath, but it's raggedy, as though I've already been sobbing, instead of being just about to.

"If it doesn't work."

"Yes?"

"If the medicine doesn't work, does that mean I'm not really sick?"

He sits forward quickly in his chair, peering sharply at me through his glasses, almost as though he is angry. And then I see as he sits back again and sighs that it isn't anger at all, but a kind of surprise, and maybe sadness, because he closes his eyes for a moment before leaning forward again, and smiles at me so kindly I might break as he says, "No, my dear. It simply means we haven't found the right medicine yet."

∞

It's late fall 1990 and no one knows what's wrong with me.

I'm in the waiting area at Beth Israel Medical Center, in a plant-filled lobby with skylighted ceilings and glass walls, sunlight brightening the institutional couches, the side tables full of year-old magazines. This is a holding space, a transitional space, an interstitial space. If this were music, it would be the kind of moment my piano teacher prizes most of all: A rest, a ritardando, a fermata. A held moment. The kind of moment players tend to hurry through, to underestimate. "Rests do not mean 'to rest,'" she tells me. "This an opportunity to stop time, prepare. Sometimes savor. Do you know what this means, stop time? You hurry, hurry. But there is time. Feel it. Rest means active. There is music even in the waiting, even in the silence."

I'm suspended here, a magazine in my lap to blend in, watching the other patients waiting. *People*, I correct myself. The other *people*. We are still people. Most of them are old. Some walk with canes, some lean on walls to steady themselves, some sit, dazed, across from me. I watch them emerge from their resting, waiting state as they hear their names called, are gathered by hospital staff, are ushered to their appointments. I watch others return from behind the doors, passing through the lobby, no longer suspended in its timelessness or affected by its atmosphere, passing through the silent sliding doors that separate this world from the other. Passing.

This is the hard part.

In my regular life, I work very hard at appearing to be well. It takes all my energy to seem as though I am not sick. I can't be sick. To be taken seriously, I must seem to be absolutely healthy, no illness, no weakness. No, not *seem* to be—I *must* be these things. I must be excellent, superhuman, even, to stand out among my music school peers, genius overachievers who have spent almost 100 percent of their young lives actively engaged in the work of being outstanding. They can sense weakness, teachers and other students alike, and the weak are dismissed. So I try my hardest to seem well. If I were to give in to this pain, this fatigue, give up and feel what I'm really feeling, I would be left behind. I must remain vigilant, appear perfectly healthy, be perfect, in order to retain my standing as a worthy competitor. In order to earn my place.

But here, at the hospital, the hypercompetence that serves me in my regular life works against me. Passing for healthy hurts my cause, marks me as a malingerer, a faker, an attention-monger. Here I must allow them to see me as vulnerable and weak, consumed by my pain, my suffering visible. I must allow myself to be sick in exactly the kinds of ways that would destroy me outside these walls.

It is hard to make that shift without thinking very seriously about the implications. If this is something I can control, this appearance or not of sickness, how deep does that go? It's true that even when passing, or trying to pass, I am struggling, I am coping with pain by denying its existence, masking its effects, even as it throbs and shoots along my nerves. But it's also true that for those moments I am successful at taming it. Could it be reasoned, then, that this mysterious pain, this mystery disease, is, in fact, something entirely under my control? And if it is, then I am faced with even more damning questions. Why, then, can't I just control it, make it stop forever? If it's true that I could make it stop forever and that I'm not making it stop forever, then have I actively chosen to be like this? Is it serving me in some way, is it useful to me somehow? Am I choosing to be sick? Is it easier to be sick than it is to fail?

I bat these questions away, send them to mix into the swirling abyss of this nonspecific, ever-shifting pain. They are too terrifying to contemplate. Because: Why would I choose something so awful? But also: What if I have?

Finally it is my turn, my name is called, other people's heads turn to watch me go. I wonder what it is they think I'm here for, how serious they think my condition is, how sick they think I am. If they think I'm sick at all.

Dr. Emily greets me and leads me to a large exam room, where two other doctors are waiting for us. She points me to a chair and makes the introductions, and then I wait, unsure of how to perform for my audience. I reflexively want to be my trying-not-to-be-in-pain self, so as to impress the doctors with my competence, my seriousness, my reliability, the way I try to with my teachers at school. But I know this may work against me.

Also, I am afraid. After holding back the pain for so long, working so hard to appear as though it doesn't affect me, if I actually relax my guard, start to let it in—I'm afraid I won't be strong enough to fight it again when I need to, when I leave this room and go back to my world.

"Can you just walk us through the timeline?" asks one of the doctors, a youngish guy with glasses and a receding hairline.

"The timeline," I repeat.

"Yes, when this all first started, everything you can remember."

June 28, 1990, 3:27 P.M. That's when the pain started. I know, because I wrote it down. But I can't tell them that. It's too absurdly precise. Suspiciously precise.

"Well, the pain first started around late June of this year," I say.

They all make note of that and return their gazes to me, expectantly.

"I had been practicing piano for about an hour—"

"She's a classical pianist," Dr. Emily interjects. Some murmurs of approval, more sounds of pens on paper. Dr. Emily nods at me to continue.

"Normally I practice for three or four hours before my hands get tired, or before I take a break. But I'd only been practicing for an hour, and I noticed my hands feeling really achy. So I massaged them for a few minutes and went back to practicing."

It was impossible to explain to them the slow creep of that first sensation of pain, the feeling of something being wrong but not knowing how wrong it would be, the retroactive sense of foreboding that accompanies the memory, knowing now that that unassuming moment—a random ache, a pause—was the start of something endless. I've retraced my steps hundreds of times, thinking back to how I could have possibly willed it on myself, that dawning moment of pain.

"But soon I noticed the aching feeling spreading up my arms and all the way to my elbows."

"So, both hands? Both arms?" This question from the older doctor. "The pain was symmetrical?"

"Not exactly," I say. "I mean, yes, both arms were affected. But it wasn't like they were mirror images of each other. They both hurt, but . . . maybe not necessarily in exactly the same specific spots. I don't know. It was kind of just all over. It's hard to remember."

I don't want to remember. But I keep remembering, hunting through the memories for clues, even when I don't want to, even when doctors aren't asking me to. It's difficult to think back further than that day in June, so that's where I start, each time, with the pain blooming from my hands. I limit my scope. It becomes a refrain in my head, a place I visit, a sequence of events I can understand because I've retold it to myself so many times.

"So the pain was in your arms," Dr. Emily prompted.

"Yes, up to my elbows. So I stopped practicing and lay in bed writing a letter, hoping the pain would stop. But instead it began spreading even more: up my arms, over my shoulders, and down my back, even to my legs and feet."

I don't tell them how I read his letter over and over, this kind-of-but-maybe-not boyfriend's letter, his words seeming like boyfriend words—"I'm sorry, I love you, I swear I do, I'll be different, I'll be better, I swear"—crying while the pain stole over me, how the pain seemed to spread like ink from the pen in my hand to the rest of my body as I wrote my response to him.

"I tried to sleep, but I felt the pain moving all over my body, until my whole body was encased in pain. My face, the top of my head, my neck. All the way to my feet. It felt like shin splints, but all over. Like I could feel my bones, but it wasn't only in my bones. Just this kind of bone-deep pain."

The doctors nod. "And then?"

"Somehow I managed to fall asleep, and when I woke up, it was a day and a half later."

"So you slept for more than 24 hours," the older doctor says.

"Yes."

"And were you still in pain when you woke up?" the younger doctor asks.

I remember the confusion as the pain dawned on me again, after all that blissful pain-free time asleep, the way my father looked at me quizzically when I emerged from my room, the way I held out my hands wordlessly and began to cry, unable to explain what was happening.

"When I first woke up, for a few minutes I didn't feel any pain at all, and I thought I must have dreamed everything. But within five minutes of waking up, the pain was back. And it's been here ever since."

The doctors exchange some glances, scribble some more notes.

"Okay," Dr. Emily says, nodding and smiling at me.

"So, can you remember, was there anything unusual that happened, health-wise, preceding this pain?" the younger doctor asks.

"What do you mean?"

"Like, had you been sick recently, before you noticed the pain starting? Had you been under a lot of stress?"

A nervous feeling settles in my stomach, and I recross my legs. I will not tell them, they cannot blame this on stress, on my being young, on my being female, on my being stupid.

"Well, I mean, before I left school I had a pretty bad flu or something."

It was the day of my sophomore recital, I was so feverish I couldn't function. A friend brought me Tylenol Cold, cough drops, nylons, helped me get dressed.

"And did you see a doctor for that?"

I shrug. "I mean, no. I had a fever, sore throat, swollen glands. It just seemed like a usual thing. Except it took forever to go away."

"What do you mean by that?" asks Dr. Emily. This may be the first time I've revealed this detail to her, the weird flu that never ended.

"Just that, I mean, even after my throat wasn't sore anymore, I still kind of felt like my glands were swollen all the time, and I kind of just always had a low-grade fever."

Frowning, scribbling.

"And when did that start?"

May 14, 1990. Four days before I turned nineteen. A week before the end of school.

"I don't remember," I say. "Sometime around the end of the semester. Right before I went home."

I will not tell them, I cannot tell them, about my not-boyfriend, about the games, about his cruelty, about the fight. About that night before I left for the summer. I trust Dr. Emily, but I can't shake the suspicion that these doctors are here to doubt me, probe me, to dissect me, to take me apart until I am too small to feel anything else but pain anymore. To blame me. But I won't confess. I will not be blamed. I will not reveal my secrets.

The doctors confer among themselves for a moment, and then Dr. Emily says, "Excuse us for a moment, please," and they leave the room.

I bring my knees up to my chest and hug them to me. It feels good to move. My shins ache, my arms ache, and when I rest my head on my knees I have to fight the urge to sleep. But I close my eyes for a moment, feel my chest rise and fall with my breath.

Dr. Emily pokes her head in the door and comes back into the room, and I unwind myself back into a normal sitting position. "So, we're going to get that blood draw today," she says. Hands in her pockets. White coat floating around her, looking too large for her.

"Do you really think I'm sick?" I ask.

A look of surprise flits across her face, but then she is back to her Dr. Emily countenance, centered and friendly and professional.

"We're all taking this seriously. Of course. You're in good hands, don't worry."

I'm grateful for her reassurance. But mostly I'm glad.

I passed.

⌀

It is winter 1990 and no one knows what's wrong with me.

Dr. Emily leans in to listen to my heart and her white coat falls open a little. Her dress is flowery, but still professional—she still seems like a doctor—and yet seeing it is startling. Proof of her humanity, her existence outside the exam room, outside the confines of her role as my doctor. She adjusts the stethoscope and moves a little closer to me, leaning even more, and I feel her belly brush my knee.

"Sorry," she says, laughing a little, gesturing to her stomach. "I keep forgetting about this thing."

I am confused for a moment, and then she stands back, her hands cradling her stomach in a suddenly familiar way, and I realize: She is pregnant. My shame is twofold: How have I not noticed this until now? And: How soon will she be leaving me, fleeing with relief from my case to care for her own, far-more-straightforward patient?

I stammer my way through the things I know people are supposed to say upon learning of someone's pregnancy, the congratulations, the due date question, but my heart is racing, the blood rushing in my ears. In a few months, she will be gone, and then who will see me? Who will see the proof of *my* humanity?

Who will believe me?

She is talking, I realize, and so I do my best to stay present, pay attention somehow, even though it feels like she has opened up a chasm beneath the exam table and I am falling through the floor.

". . . maternity leave, but as I said, that won't start until mid-January. And don't worry, I've been meeting with the whole team to make sure everyone's on the same page. I actually presented you at grand rounds last week. You're quite the conundrum. I also had a nice talk with the rheumatologist. He had a few thoughts about what might be going on with you, even though the blood work didn't pan out. You're still taking the medication he prescribed?"

"Yes," I say, "though mostly all I can feel are side effects. It hasn't helped with the pain or anything." Drowsiness, as he predicted. And an added layer of fog during the daytime. A kind of numbness. But not enough.

"Hmm," she says. "And by this point it really should be working, if it was going to work for you at all."

I see a flash of his kindly face, a lurch of my stomach as I remember his words. *My dear. It simply means we haven't found the right medicine yet.*

She sighs as she closes my file and sits back on the round rolling exam-room chair. "I'll be honest. This is a mystery. I don't want to say we're hitting a dead end, but. We're getting close."

I'm the dead end. I am dead. No: This is my life, this pain, this fog, this endless aching, this endless exhaustion. It would be better if I were dead. Dr. Emily wouldn't be here looking so sad, cradling her baby belly, shaking her head over me, wasting her time. I'm sure she'd much rather be home, decorating a nursery, folding tiny clothes into drawers, focusing on the life she will be birthing, not this dead end, not me.

"So that's it? There's no answer? We're just done?" I try but it's impossible not to cry, not to have my stupid ineffectual tears leaking down to my nose, my lips.

She rolls closer to the exam table and puts a hand on my knee. "Of course not. We're going to keep looking. We're going get to the bottom of this. Or do our best to try to, anyway."

I bet she will be a good mother. I can see her, in her Dr. Emily clothes, her white coat and stethoscope, holding a tiny baby, soothing it with quiet sounds and gentle rocking. Putting a Band-Aid on a skinned knee. Reading a bedtime story while idly caressing a toddler's hair as they lie in bed together. But just imagining this opens up a yawing need, a clawing at a tender place, that makes me feel like I might cry forever, so I squeeze the flesh of my right hand between my thumb and finger with my left hand and try to push it down, all of it, everything.

"So. Moving forward," she says. "When you come next week, I'll introduce you to the doctor who will be taking over for me while I'm on maternity leave. And I'd also like you to start seeing Dr. Cohen."

"Who's that? Another specialist?"

She hesitates, and then says, gently. "He's a psychiatrist."

I look up at the ceiling. Maybe gravity will keep the tears inside my eyes. "So you're giving up on me."

"No, I am most definitely not," she says, standing. I feel her hands on my shoulders, her belly grazing my knees. "I promise you I'm not. Dr. Cohen is merely one part of the team, one part of the overall treatment plan we're putting together here."

I wipe my eyes, head down now, forcing her hands off my shoulders.

"Look, there's no reason why you shouldn't get some support while you're going through all this," she says. "It's got to be stressful for you, feeling so sick, being so worried about what might be wrong with you while also dealing with the symptoms you have. Doesn't it make sense to talk to someone about it? And possibly be treated with medication that might help you cope? That's all Dr. Cohen is here, another piece of the puzzle, to support you while we figure out what's wrong."

"It sounds like," I say, and now I don't even bother trying to keep it together, appear sane, be the good patient. I am crying the kind of embarrassing, heaving sobs that make it impossible to talk. There is snot running down my face, my eyes hurt from crying. But I don't care. Everything hurts, everything is pain, I don't have the energy to pretend like I'm okay anymore. "It sounds like you just think I'm crazy. Like that's why I'm sick. I'm just crazy. That's what you want me to admit, right? That I'm crazy? And then I can just go away and stop bothering everybody. Is that it?"

I wipe my nose with my sleeve and look up to see Dr. Emily's eyes bright with her own tears. But she blinks quickly, pulls it together.

"No," she says, her voice quiet but steady. "That's not it."

For a moment the only sounds in the room are my sniffing, my breath catching on dying sobs as I try to calm myself down.

"I don't think you're crazy. I think you're in pain. And I don't know why. And, while we try to figure it out, I want you to have someone to talk to about the pain you're in. Maybe that's all you'll do with Dr. Cohen is talk. Or maybe he'll prescribe you something that might help you cope with your pain level. That's for the two of you to figure out together."

I nod my head. It feels like we're done here. Like everything is done.

"Oh!" She exclaims. I glance up and see her looking at me apologetically, a hand on her belly. "I'm sorry—the baby just kicked. It surprised me. I don't know that I'll ever get used to it."

"The kicking?"

"The idea that there's actually a person in there." She turns back to the rolling chair, picks up my file. "So amazing, the secret things bodies can do."

"Yes," I say. But I'm not thinking about the baby blindly moving and turning inside her. I'm thinking about my pain, the deep, black ache of it, how I picture it like tentacles, inexorably squeezing my body, wrapping itself around my bones, choking me, relentlessly growing inside me, with a consciousness all its own, a biological imperative to exist that is directly at odds with my own existence. How I am its host, how somehow I have nurtured this, willed it into being, allowed it to flourish inside me, given it life.

∞

It's late winter 1990 and no one knows what's wrong with me.

The room is dark and chilly, and I'm dismayed when the tech tosses me a hospital gown and yanks the privacy curtain around me so that I can change. I'm already so freezing.

I gown up, leaving my socks on, and push back the curtain.

"Just a few more minutes," he says, squinting at his computer monitor, adjusting a piece of machinery.

I wrap the hospital gown tighter around me.

"You okay?" he asks. He's frowning at me as though I've done something wrong.

"Just cold," I say.

"No, I mean, what are you in for?"

I don't understand, and he looks exasperated before turning back to the monitor.

"Why are you having this done, what are you sick with," he says, as if that makes it easier for me.

"I—" I begin. "I don't know. That's why we're doing it."

"You don't know?" Now he seems outright disgusted. He mutters something under his breath and says, "This is a very expensive test, you know? It's not just a thing you do to rule stuff out."

I can feel my throat constricting, my eyes burning with the beginnings of tears. I focus on the ground, on my feet in their whitish-pinkish socks, survivors of some long-ago laundry incident, on the coldness of the cement floor beneath them.

"I'm here because my doctor ordered it. That's all I know."

He mutters something under his breath again, but louder this time, loud enough for me to almost hear it. *Fucking waste of my time.*

"Excuse me?" I look up at him, staring at him directly, daring him to repeat himself.

"It's just, you look fine to me," he says. "The people that usually get sent down here?" He shakes his head. "It's no joke."

"Yeah, well," I say. "I'm not laughing."

Finally he guides me to the platform, another cold place, where I am to waste his time by lying on a wide table, which turns out to be even harder and colder than I anticipated, even with the thin blanket he provided as cushion. My teeth are chattering and my tears are running down the side of my face as I look up. Above me is a light so bright it obscures everything. The tech is now a dark shape who busily moves things above me, beside me. I hear the whir and clank of machines, but everything is that bright light, and the sound of my own teeth hitting together.

"It's very important that you don't move." His head butts in front of the light as he leans over the table, and now he is a dark-green human-shaped thing looming above me, a corona of spotlight shimmering around him. "No teeth chattering. No more crying."

"Okay," I say, but it makes my teeth chatter more, my nose run.

I close my eyes as the machine above me comes to life, a camera scanning me for abnormalities, hunting for information. A fucking waste of time.

∽

It's spring 1991 and no one knows what's wrong with me.

Every week I am given a new potential diagnosis: lupus, multiple sclerosis, Epstein-Barr virus, parvovirus, cytomegalovirus. None of these pan out, except for my positive results for Epstein-Barr virus and cytomegalovirus, but those are so common and unlikely to be the culprits behind my endless pain that they are dismissed, and the doctors have exhausted all the tests they can think to give.

"It's a puzzle," Dr. Emily, fresh off maternity leave, tells me. "I've never been stumped like this before. I feel terrible that we haven't been able to help you."

She suggests that this may be what's called a somatoform pain disorder. In other words: psychosomatic.

"That's not exactly what it means," she clarifies. "What somatoform pain disorder means is that there's an idiopathic component to what you're experiencing."

Idiopathic. *Idio*, meaning "one's own" or "private," plus -*pathic*, from *pathos*, "suffering," "something endured." My own private suffering. Meaning this pain is something that has been invented— curated, nurtured, caused, allowed to flourish—entirely by me.

Dr. Emily hastens to assure me that people with somatoform pain disorder experience very real pain—it's just that the pain lacks a discernible physical cause.

This is the psychiatrist's fault, I know it. Or, rather, my fault: I didn't bother trying to perform for him, to be a good patient. I was angry, and defensive, and resistant to the process, even though I could see him understanding this, writing down "angry," "defensive," "resistant to the process."

"So, what," I'd said, at our first meeting, "I'm supposed to sit here and tell you about my dreams and fall in love with you?"

"Is that what you think is supposed to happen?" he countered.

"Well, isn't that the cliché about psychiatrists?"

"That patients form attachments to their therapists? Sure, that can be part of the therapeutic process." He sat neutrally in his chair, his face open and expressionless, a blank canvas awaiting my projection.

"I think it's a story psychiatrists tell themselves to make themselves feel better," I said.

He nodded. "Is that something you ever find yourself doing? Telling yourself stories to make yourself feel better?"

I felt caught for a moment, but I said, "I'm not going to fall for this. I'm not going to do what everyone wants me to do."

"And what do you think it is that everyone wants you to do?"

"Prove that this 'illness' is all in my head. That it's not real, that I'm not sick, I'm just a crazy person."

"Do you think 'crazy people' aren't really sick?"

"Look, that's why they sent me to you," I said. "It's the option of last resort. They want you to agree with them that I'm just crazy, and then they can write me off, problem solved, oh, she's a teenager, a musician, a girl—isn't that the definition of crazy? Being female? I don't want to be sick. I didn't choose this, I didn't decide to be in pain all the time and tired and miserable, I didn't make this happen. But I want them to find something actually wrong with me, because otherwise. . ."

He waited for me to continue, and then when it was clear that I couldn't, he said, "You don't want to be sick, because of course who would choose to be sick. And yet you want for there to be something identifiably wrong, and you want a 'real' medical diagnosis, so as to justify all of this time and expense and pain and effort, because otherwise, you feel, you are just 'crazy' and beyond help and entirely at fault. Do I have this right?"

"Yes," I said, blinking back tears.

"That is a difficult story to be telling yourself."

And yet, as I see it now, the story seems to be that Dr. Emily and her team think I am making this up. They recommend more medication—a low dose of Elavil, an antidepressant—and weekly meetings with a social worker in addition to monthly check-ins with the psychiatrist; but no longer will I be needing regular appointments with Dr. Emily. She has exhausted her medical expertise on me, and there is no more she can do. Dr. Emily stops me at the door before I leave.

"I tried, kiddo, I really did," she says. "This case keeps me up at night. I wish I had something better to tell you."

⁓

It's late spring 1991 and no one knows what's wrong with me, but now I have the catchall diagnosis of "chronic fatigue syndrome," even though my defining symptom is still pain, the feeling of shin splints all over my body. Chronic fatigue syndrome can cause this, the doctors say. The doctors also say this is sometimes called "the yuppie flu," as it tends to hit "type-A" personalities, driven people, people who might work long hours and push themselves really hard and one day get sick with some kind of virus or flu and push themselves through it and do a recital anyway even though they have a 102-degree fever, and then somehow their bodies never get the message to stop fighting it. And so their bodies fight themselves, remain in a perpetual state of fighting off that flu. The swollen glands, the constant low-grade fever, the body aches: those are symptoms of the body fighting off a thing, not necessarily the thing itself. The pain, the constant pain, is my body fighting itself.

I'm told to rest. To take medicine. To slow down. To not push myself. I'm given Prozac, which keeps me awake for three days straight; then Zoloft, which makes me gain twenty pounds in a month. I take a powerful antiviral medication five times a day. I keep going. I keep sleeping. I keep hurting.

I cry one day during my piano lesson, exhausted by Beethoven's Waldstein sonata and frustrated and tired. "It isn't fair," I manage to choke out. But my piano teacher isn't having it. "Nothing is fair," she says. "Music isn't fair. Beethoven isn't fair." She waits for me to stop crying, wipe the tears from my face. For a moment, I think she might be about to offer some words of comfort, or maybe wisdom. But all she says is, "Play."

∽

It's spring 1992, graduation, just a few days before my twenty-first birthday. I am still aching, still sick with this mystery disease. I am valedictorian.

I return home to Southern California, prepare to start graduate school in San Francisco in a few months. I compete in one of the annual state piano competitions, playing Ravel and Beethoven through aching hands and forearms. I win.

$\backsim$

It's fall 1993, and I am twenty-two. I'm studying at the San Francisco Conservatory, working part time as an editor at a news wire service, seeing a chronic fatigue specialist named, aptly, Dr. Rest.

Rests do not mean "to rest," my old piano teacher's voice reminds me. *This an opportunity to stop time, prepare.* I try to stop time. I take direction from Dr. Rest. I take the herbal "energy" medicine I will understand only later to be straight ephedra, soon to be banned by the FDA. I drink chlorophyll, I boil twigs and bark. I sleep on a tower of soft foam mattress toppers, my bones cushioned, my pain met with acceptance instead of resistance. I try to sleep when I am tired, eat when I am hungry, accommodate this pain rather than fight it. I try to prepare.

$\backsim$

It's fall 1995. Dr. Rest has quit medicine and moved to the Midwest to pursue his love of regional musical theater. I have quit his medicine and moved east to pursue a relationship with Gil, who seems to love me despite my pain. We are married. In the days I work in New York City; in the evenings I teach and practice on the grand piano he bought me as an engagement ring. Soon I will begin to prepare for a recital at Carnegie Hall's Weill Recital Hall. I plan my repertoire, outline my practice schedule, use a pencil to notate on the score those places where I must be mindful of resting, of using the time I have, or creating time where there is none, to rest, regroup, prepare, sometimes savor. I'm no longer seeing any doctors, no longer taking any medicine. My pain is now occasional, transient, normal: the acceptable pain of stubbing a toe or getting a paper cut or otherwise being a human in the everyday world. Sometimes my body will flare with fever when I have an ordinary winter flu, and my bones will ache in that familiar way, and I'll think, *Okay, here we go, it's back.* But then the body aches fade as the fever fades, and I return to a state of normalcy, the kind of pain-free experience of life I'd worried might be lost to me forever. My body has learned to stop fighting itself. I'm learning to stop fighting myself. Am I better? Am I cured?

∽

It's early summer 1996, and I'm no longer in pain. I am reading a book called *Osler's Web*, a look at the late 1980s/early 1990s chronic fatigue syndrome epidemic, and I learn that I'm far from the only person to have suffered from the disease, whose proper name is myalgic encephalomyelitis, and far from the only person to have been told her pain is all in her head. The book reads like a novel, a medical mystery complete with heroes like the dogged immunologist Elaine DeFreitas of the Wistar Institute, and villains like the CDC, which allegedly deliberately mismanaged the over 150 million taxpayer dollars marked for research into the disease beginning in 1988. But what strikes me at the time is a paragraph about the prognosis of CFS/ME patients, which says that people either seemed to recover within about five years, or not at all.

I shiver as I realize: It's almost exactly five years to the day since the pain stole over my fingers and hands and ached its way into my body.

I shiver as I realize: I'm one of the lucky ones.

The precise cause of spontaneous spinal CSF leaks remains largely unknown. . . . A history of a more or less trivial traumatic event preceding the onset of symptoms can be elicited in about one third of patients, suggesting a role for mechanical factors as well.

—Wouter I. Schievink, "Spontaneous Spinal Cerebrospinal Fluid Leaks and Intracranial Hypotension," *JAMA*, 2006

15

July 2015

When I was in graduate school, I lived in San Francisco near Ocean Beach, it was like permanently being in a 1940s movie. Dark, foggy, cold; everything practically in black and white. I'd shed my layers on my way downtown, starting off on the N-Judah dressed for winter, ending up aboveground at Civic Center in my summer clothes, my music bag stuffed with the sweater, jacket, long-sleeved shirt I'd discarded as I made my way to the sunlight. On the return trip home, I could literally see the fog rolling in, marveling how it was just like the way people always say it, the fog literally rolling in. In the distance it looked like something solid, something you could part with your hands or maybe carve your way through. Every time I'd keep waiting for that moment: waiting to get there, to the solid part. But that moment never came. Instead the fog just rolled in to meet me, so stealthily I didn't realize it was all the way fully there until I found myself enveloped in it, stepping off the cable car and remembering: *Of course, it isn't solid, it isn't carvable, it's particulate, it's not a wall, it's not a door, it's the air, it's all around you.* There isn't a specific moment when you enter the fog or the fog enters you. It's just there. You don't even realize you're in the middle of it until it's too late.

That's how it is right now. The fog is rolling in. And I'm at the edge of it now, the part where I can see it's not a thing I can push against, where I can see it floating around me, swirling at my feet and obscuring everything far away, reducing the landscape to the few bright things that can penetrate the haze.

I'm back to wondering how many of my decisions are thoughtful, considered, smart thinking, and how much of it is this fog: *That shiny thing there, I can see it, it must be a good idea.* I'm wearing compression clothes, things that place pressure on my dura, sending the cerebro spinal fluid upward, helping my brain float a little, but still not as much as it needs to. I'm drinking caffeine, dilating my blood vessels, but not enough to provide the pressure I need inside my head. I have marshaled my resources to function, managing to be upright through relatives' visits, through my youngest sister's wedding, summoning my fading abilities to be present for the kids' emergencies, the day Gil moved out of the house, his father telling me it was the worst day of his life, the same day the cat escaped, or so we thought, and we printed out and hung up missing-cat posters throughout the neighborhood before finding him doing what I should have been doing: lying down, hiding, sleeping in a dark place. The only time my head doesn't hurt now is when I'm unconscious.

Awake, I'm permanently in this tipsy stage, the part where my drunk self congratulates every tangential idea it has. *Great job! Yes!*

That sounds logical! You should do that! I can talk to people, usually, if I haven't been upright too long, and I hear myself telling stories, making jokes, finding ways to be funny. It's what my drunk brain does. It's what my adolescent brain did, kicking into some gear to make me the funniest person in the room instead of the shyest or weirdest or quietest. I can gloss over things. I can make small talk. I sat down to play the piano the other day and to my surprise I found myself able to play through, almost all the way through, pieces I'd previously forgotten. I'd play through the parts I definitely still remembered and then get to the "Oops, that's gone now" part and instead—just keep on playing. It was like some kind of special bullshit ability turned on in my brain and I could just bulldoze my way through. Not perfectly, but well enough to get through it, get through the parts that had fallen out of my head and back to the other parts I still had memorized. It's all part of this brain fog/drunk brain thing, I think, this thing that takes over when my actual brain is shutting down a little bit from lack of fluid.

When it was really foggy, in the foggy part of San Francisco where I lived, if you walked far enough into the fog, it did get thicker—never an actual wall of fog you could slice through with your hands or fluff like a pillow, but thick enough so that on a dark night you couldn't even see a streetlight until you were almost directly underneath it. If you walked far enough, if you kept walking past my house in that fog, in the seemingly interminable gray mist between streetlights, eventually you'd come to a place with no lights, with a bank you'd scramble up blindly, where the ground beneath your feet grew shiftable, changeable, and the fog itself began to have a sound. And if you walked far enough, if you followed that sound, you'd find yourself walking right into the sea.

I need to have this fixed before I get there. Before I get submerged again to the point where I can't think or read or write or watch TV or have conversations. Before the things happen again where I can't feel my arms when I close my eyes, or I start crying uncontrollably if I've been standing up for five minutes, or I have panic attacks when I lie down. I don't want to be in this fog, I don't want to drown in this ocean. I want my brain back.

16

I am walking, but I don't know how. If I stop to think about it, I become baffled as to how it is possible, how my body knows what to do.

As long as I am in motion, I am distracted, the pain muted temporarily by the movement of my body through space. My head throbs, but not as much as it does when I'm standing still, and the forward momentum of my physical self as I walk lulls my brain into a kind of dull satisfaction. *I am moving, I am walking somewhere, this is what people do, I am doing it.*

At a crosswalk, I wait at the corner, understanding by sheer reflex to obey the red light, and as soon as I stand still the pain rushes back, flooding my head, a wave crashing on rocks. The base of my skull pounds and throbs, an echo of the rhythm of my walking, until the tide settles again from my standing still and the pain morphs back into its usual constant assault, bright and steady. I grip the right side of my head, pressing against the base of my skull as if to hold it in place. This is another distraction from the pain. But it's nothing that lasts, nothing that makes it go away.

The light is green but I'm still standing there. People brush past me and then I realize, *Oh, I should walk now*, and then I do. I am going to the store. Why am I going to the store? I need to go to the store. I keep walking, somehow knowing how to go to the store, and then I remember, *I need to get pasta and Benadryl and Advil and Band-Aids, that's why I'm going to the store*. The pain in my head, so steady and unceasing once I am finally standing still, now pulses with my footsteps. I'm tempted to keep walking forever, because of how painful my head feels when I stop, and yet I'm aware that the longer I am upright, the worse I feel, the less clearly I can think, the more punishing the pain becomes, the stranger the strange things are that begin to happen.

I find myself approaching the entrance to the store, and I have a fleeting sensation of both recognition and surprise. How did I get here? And yet I am here. *You did it!* My brain congratulates me, and I feel inordinately accomplished. I made it to the store, the whole way, all four blocks. My head throbs. It feels as though my whole body now pulses with the pain of it as I stand there, trying to orient myself outside the store. For a moment I feel a rush of confusion—*Why am I outside this store?*—but my body moves me forward and I walk through the automatic doors, the rush of air conditioning goose bumping my skin.

Once inside, once I'm no longer propelling myself down the street at a normal walking pace like a normal person, I'm caught by the resurgence of my pain. The base of my skull is a sharp demanding sensation that overtakes my ability to make sense of everything, of anything. There is a cacophony of information: the music in the air around me, the words in that music; the assault of illumination, the overhead lights like spotlights aimed at my cortex; the towering aisles of color, products aligned and stacked and displayed, everything competing for my attention. Three steps inside the store and I am overwhelmed. *Why am I here? How did I get here? What did I come here for again?* The pain crowds out everything, and so I begin to walk the aisles, hoping that movement will dull things again, that walking past all the organized items on the shelves will trigger a memory of what I'm there for, or remind me of what it is that I had intended to do.

Instead I find myself beginning to panic, the pain overtaking me. I can't think, and if I close my eyes, I can't feel where my left arm is in space. It's like if I close my eyes, a part of me doesn't exist anymore. If I close my eyes, all there's room for is pain. And yet my head hurts so much that closing my eyes is all I can think to do, and when I open my eyes to locate my disappearing left arm again, I realize I am crying—not because I'm upset, but because this is what happens when I'm upright for more than fifteen minutes. I have reached my limit. But I don't know what to do. I keep wandering the aisles, an empty basket in my hand—*When did you get a basket?*—tears streaming down my face, my skull aching as though my brain is trying to tunnel its way out. Eventually, the only thing that makes sense to me is to give up. I stare down at the empty basket, a part of me reminding myself that I must return it to its rightful place before I can leave. *Just find the place where the baskets live and return this one to its family*, my brain tells me, and this makes complete sense to me in the moment. And then I am walking out the door, back into the thick Philadelphia heat, my body propelling me home. *You can just come back later, when you remember what you were supposed to get,* my brain assures me. *That's a fantastic idea,* it congratulates me. And as I feel myself thinking that thought, it really does seem like a fantastic idea. It seems like something that makes sense. I should probably believe it.

I have done this before. I'll find myself in the midst of a rainy day, somehow walking, somehow having had the foresight to hold an umbrella, heading to the school to get the kids and shepherd them home, my brain congratulating me on having such a brilliant idea, for doing the things a parent is supposed to do, getting her children from school, bringing an umbrella on a rainy day. I'll find myself standing, making dinner, and discovering that we have run out of butter, and then walking the two minutes to the corner store and remembering once I get there that I was there to buy butter, like a normal person who buys butter at the corner store when they run out of butter. These are normal things a person should do. But I should not be doing these things. I should be lying in bed, flat, preserving what little cerebrospinal fluid I have, allowing gravity to help it pool in my head, support my brain, keep it even slightly cushioned. I should not be standing, the fluid draining, my brain sinking, bruising, a fish out of water, dying. But I am overtaken sometimes by the desire to accomplish things, to organize, to make things right, to power through, to be okay, and after lying flat for twelve hours, eighteen hours, twenty-four hours, I feel the rush of overconfidence, the boost of having my brain irrigated even some-what. And so I find myself in the kitchen, for instance, standing, at least for brief periods, preparing snacks, or wiping counters, or feeding cats, or making dinner, or putting things away, my arms and hands moving like someone else's arms and hands, my body moving through the motions like a remote-controlled robot, an artificial intelligence passing almost as human.

I am aware that these are bad ideas, and yet I'm so frustrated by being flat, so helpless with pain, so frustrated and trapped-feeling that I am energized by the sheer rebelliousness of these bad ideas, which are not actually bad at all (or even legitimate *ideas*, in the true sense of the word) for a normal person. When I am flat, and lulled by the presence of a little fluid between my brain and skull,

I am as fooled as I am when I am walking and in motion. The diversion of a momentary respite from the worst of things fills me with misplaced confidence, and for a moment I am full of plans, full of thoughts, full of guilt and shame and terror, full of ambition to get out of bed and back into my real life. Full of resistance to the notion that this could possibly be, at this moment and maybe for the foreseeable future, my real life.

I could ask someone else to go to the store. I could ask someone else to pick up my children on a rainy day. And I do, as much as it makes this my real life to ask favors of other people, as much as it is an admission of defeat to acknowledge my helplessness, the fact that I need things, that I have needs, that I need help, I do. But I still keep trying. I stand up for longer than I should. I make a rare attempt at dinner and an even rarer appearance at the dinner table with my kids, sitting with them even as I can feel myself crying from being up, feel myself getting dumber the longer I'm up, all of us laughing at the way I forget words, or say wrong words, or mean a thing I couldn't articulate, or articulate a thing I didn't mean. And then I retreat again to the darkness of my room, shrouded in curtains to block out the light, my bed piled with pillows I can't use as I lie flat, flat, flat to counteract having been upright for so long.

One day, seduced by the idea that I need to go to the store again, ignoring the fact that I could easily order what I need from an app on my phone, compelled by the immediacy, the fantasy of being able to get the thing I needed by myself, without help, I decide to go to the store. But this time, I come up with what my brain assures me is a fool-proof plan: I will write myself a shopping list. This way, even if I find myself disoriented when I get there, butting up against the fifteen-minute time limit of my ability to think with admittedly limited clarity, I will have information at the ready, alerting me to what my purpose is. I would not return home empty-handed.

Genius! My brain congratulates me as I open up the Notes app on my phone and type instructions for my future self.

I walk to the store the way people talk about driving on auto-pilot, the car taking you where you need to go even though you yourself are daydreaming, or talking to a passenger, or otherwise not thinking about your destination. I make it there, and, predictably, feel the usual overwhelming rush of information overload. The lights, the exhausting amount of information to take in, the vertigo of so many products on so many shelves in so many aisles. The pain is overwhelming and feels like a punishment—*How brazen of you, how prideful, how foolish of you to think that you could do this*—and as if on cue I feel the tears beginning to stream down my face, my left arm disappearing.

But then my brain remembers: *You wrote yourself a note!* I take out my phone, triumphant and relieved and congratulating myself for having been so forward-thinking as to provide such crucial information for Future Me, who is now Present Me, crying in the middle of a Walgreens, unsure why she's there in the first place—only to open the app and be confronted with the truth of what I had written. I stare at it, trying to comprehend it, for surely I had been more thorough, I remember being thorough, I remember writing myself the information I was sure I'd need once I made it to the store. But no matter how long I stare at it, no matter how many times I close and open the app, my note to self, my shopping list, contains only two words.

"Get stuff."

Later I will tell this story as a funny story. It turned out to be, in fact, my kids' favorite story from this time in our lives. *Get stuff!* How hilarious! How dumb! How useless! And later it will become funnier to me, or rather I will be able to appreciate more how funny it was, this example of the ways all of us fool ourselves, the ways in which we think we are competent, the ways in which our own view of ourselves is so limited in perspective and scope, the ways in which we all struggle to prepare ourselves and cope, and yet how misplaced our confidence is, how limited our abilities.

At the moment, however, it is crushing. Humiliating. Specific to only me. Even though I can't think clearly enough to fully think through what is happening, what had just happened, I'm able to fully experience the confusion, the panic, the terror of being unable to think, the shame of having thought so poorly. I'm merely going through the motions of thinking, going through the motions of being a person who can go to the store, a person who can make lists of things she needs at the store and then go to the store and then get those things and not have any of that be confusing or strange or even remarkable in any way, going through the motions of being me. But I'm not me. At least not the me I've been able to rely on for as long as I'd been alive, not a me I recognize.

I walk home crying, and not only from being upright too long. "Get stuff."

Who was the me who had written myself that note? Who was the me who had thought it had made sense? Who was the me who walked to the store? Who was the me who couldn't remember why she was at the store in the first place? Had this me always been like this? Am I only seeing now what a fiction this is, this self that is apparently assembled, context-less and free-floating? Is this me my brain? And if it is, who am I when that brain isn't working?

My best thoughts were incomplete thoughts. Useless messages from a self I didn't recognize. The me who was Me—my consciousness, my self, the thing that used to be able to understand context and purpose and thought and story—was somehow dampened, muted, held prisoner by the me who was the rest of my brain, the me who regulated my breathing and got signals from nerve endings and oversaw the beating of my heart and the circulation of my blood and the production of my cerebrospinal fluid, and the me who could walk to the store or make dinner if I needed to or babble like a drunk person in response to questions without actually thinking or understanding or even making sense.

I walk home, crying, defeated, and return to the darkness of my room, to my bed, to the comfort and humiliation of being flat. The hubris of thinking that I could think! The cockiness of assuming I could complete an errand! I lie in shame, staring at the ceiling, podcast voices interrupting each other in the background with forced banter, until finally I begin to feel myself shifting into sleep, the sensation of pain merging with the sensation of slipping away, the voices becoming more and more indistinct, less identifiable as people speaking words. And as I start to feel the me who is still me fully fall away, my brain whispers to me: *Shampoo and conditioner!* My phone is too far away to write it down, but I feel my brain confidently telling me, *That's okay, You'll remember it, you can go back to the store tomorrow. Just make a list.*

17

August 2015

The thought saunters in, as all of my thoughts do these days: a plain fact, casually registering in my consciousness, free of judgment aside from a friendly welcoming impulse. My brain is now perpetually agreeable to thoughts. My brain perpetually says yes, acknowledging thoughts with pleasant surprise, without discrimination. And so I'm not disturbed when the thought appears. Instead I welcome it the way my brain now welcomes all ideas, with a moment of feigned recognition, the way you might improvise delight at parties when being introduced to someone you don't remember but surely should. *Ah! Hello! Of course!* That's how I reacted when the thought made itself known, when I sat up in bed, the whole world a flat and unceasing sensation of pain, and felt some part of me think: *Remember, if it gets really bad, you can just take all of your medicine at once and kill yourself.*

I have wanted to die twice before. Well, *wanted* is a strong word. Perhaps better to say: Twice I have realized it was an appealing option. The first time was in the midst of labor with Emi, the pain so wrenching and overwhelming that I found myself having reached a place of surrender, thinking *I understand now; if it's my time, it's my time; I'm okay with this, I can go now.* And then suddenly the pain gave way to progress and I emerged on the other side of it into a new plane of existence, for sure, but not the noncorporeal one I had, for one surprisingly peaceful moment, imagined.

The second time contained no such grace.

In the bathroom, I open the medicine cabinet. There are easily fifteen bottles there, medication I have been prescribed but, for the most part, have not taken. Powerful prophylactic antibiotics, for the surgery I ended up not having. Painkillers that were barely capable of wounding my pain, let alone killing it. Migraine pills (which did nothing), neuro meds (which made me feel worse), a couple of steroids left over from a weeklong course that didn't help me think any clearer, but did make me feel as though I could. Motivated and energized, but still lacking lucidity, this mostly resulted in bold, ill-conceived home-improvement projects, and ill-advised impulse Amazon purchases, which would surprise me later when they arrived as if of their own accord.

Early on in my internet research, trying to learn more about CSF leaks and my strange constant headache, I came across an interview with George Clooney, in which he mentioned the strange constant headache of his own CSF leak, and reported that the pain was so bad he wanted to die. I remember feeling relief, as though his admission finally legitimized my own pain. "Even George Clooney wants to kill himself. And he's George Clooney!" I wrote in the text I sent to my husband.

It would be easy enough to do. Probably any one of these bottles, taken all at once, would be enough to make all of this stop forever. It's not a terrifying thought at all. It reminds me of the acceptance I felt in the midst of that intractable labor pain, in that it feels strangely comforting. *I'm okay with this, I can go now.* I close the mirrored cabinet and know that my mirror self and I have come to an understanding. For a moment, we both feel the relief of knowing there's a way out.

"Shouldn't you be dead?" a friend texts. "I mean, if your brain isn't working?"

It's a fair question, and I know the answer, but it floats away from me, a note in a bottle, bobbing in the ocean. My brain works well enough to keep going, I explain. It does the basic things it's supposed to do. I can breathe, I can walk, I can talk, I can function physically, aside from the small weirdnesses I have begun to notice: the way that lying on my left side brings on a panic attack, my heart flubbing weirdly in my chest, a strange rush of adrenaline burbling inside me; the way that once I've been upright for too long, my eyes stream tears, but not from sadness; the way everything feels odd and disconnected, as though my body is moving of its own accord, without my brain to tell it what I want it to do or where I want it to go.

It's like being very, very, very drunk, I explain. I have never actually been very, very, very drunk, I have only ever been tipsy; but that is what this feels like, except more so, the whole world tipping over while my mouth still moves, my legs still walk, the way a drunk person can talk and walk and think that they are fine.

"So you're fine, then," this friend says.

I am not. But also, I am. Because he has a point. I'm not in a coma. I'm not paralyzed. I'm not on life support. I'm just in pain, stuck in bed, my brain in a fog.

"Everyone feels foggy like that," he says. "Part of aging."

"You're right," I say. "That's true."

My brain agrees with everything.

This must be a coping mechanism, this agreement, a small part of me thinks from way back in the recesses of my brain. It's as though the me who is Me is just a tiny seed of a me, swathed in cotton, far, far away, and every once in a while I can hear some kind of distant echo of a thought that makes sense. But of course these thoughts will make sense: My brain is eminently agreeable, and so it welcomes all thoughts with the same dumb enthusiasm. *A coping mechanism! Yes! Brilliant!*

The second time I wanted to die also involved my children. It was not the pain of deliverance, though, not the surrender of acceptance. It was the powerlessness all parents are confronted with at one time or another. The guilt of a split-second of inattention. The general parental agony of being unable to protect your child from the harm inherent in the world, and the specific parental agony of having been responsible for it.

Nate was three, Emi was six. It was President's Day, the children home from school. I was getting ready to take them out to some activity, to break up the monotony of the morning inside our small apartment. Nate and I were in the bathroom, he washing his hands, me putting on makeup. It was a normal day.

How many times did I go over this sequence of events after what followed? How many times did I live these moments?

He slapped his hands on the towel in a simulacrum of drying them, and ran off to retrieve his cars, which he'd been in the middle of racing up and down the bed of the treadmill that stood in our living room. I leaned into the mirror to better see what as I was doing as I put on my eyeliner, and I heard a strange, loud grunt. It was a sound not unlike other sounds I'd heard my children make when they fought—and yet somehow immediately I knew this was not a fighting grunt, not a grunt about someone hogging space on the table for coloring or someone taking someone else's favorite car.

"Nate?" I called from the bathroom, still looking at myself, frozen in the mirror. But then I ran, because everything in my body felt wrong, a sickening rush of adrenaline flooding me with panic.

I ran around the corner from the bathroom to find him slumped against the living room wall, behind the treadmill, near the couch, his mouth open, his eyes wide. As I ran to him, calling his name, his eyes widened even more, and then rolled back in his head, and then he seemed to fade away, the life falling away from him, before his body started shaking with seizures. He gripped his toy car in one hand as he seized up, his other hand flailing near the extension cord on the floor behind the couch. *Wet hands. Cord.*

I scooped him up, and he was dead weight, his body limp for a moment. I laid him on the couch and he continued to seize, his eyelids fluttering. Emi, too, was fluttering, alighting from one couch to another like a nervous bird, panicking, asking "Is he dead, is he dead?", over and over while I kept shouting, "Oh god, oh god, Nate," as I tried to revive him. He wasn't breathing. "Is he dead?" Emi screamed, and I told her no, but to myself I said *Not yet,* and as I leaned over his face, listening for breath, Emi jumping and panicking in my peripheral vision, I swore that if he was dead, I would kill myself.

Somehow I found the phone, somehow I dialed *11, 811, then 711, then finally 911, somehow I screamed our address over the phone and told them to hurry while they told me to calm down. Then it was Emi telling me to call Daddy, Emi telling me she was scared, that she was going to run for help. Nate turning blue, turning gray, shaking and shaking. Me trying to rescue-breathe for him, me turning him over onto his side and hearing him finally take a breath. The 911 person telling me to try to stand him up, but Nate was too limp, me trying, Nate falling, me dropping the phone, me carrying him to the front door, realizing that Emi was nowhere. A man showing up telling me he'd found Emi on the stairs, she was too scared to take the elevator by herself, that he'd told the front desk to call an ambulance, that Emi had told this man that she had just watched her little brother die in my arms.

Finally the paramedics arrived, rushing in, wanting to know what happened, but of course I didn't totally know, I had been in the bathroom, staring at myself in the mirror, and Emi couldn't tell them: In her six-year-old version of events she had seen him explode in lightning bolts and then fade into nothingness before he died. But he wasn't dead. He was moaning, making sounds, starting to open his eyes, saying "Mommy" as they lifted him onto the gurney.

"I don't want to ride in the ambulance, I want to stay here in case Nate dies, I don't want to see him die again," Emi told me, but we had to ride in the ambulance, even though it was scary, even though it seemed like Nate might die again as he vomited and passed out.

Once we got to the ER, Nate was conscious, but crying, screaming, trying to talk but unable to talk, unable to focus. Agitated. Emi wanted to know that he was okay, but was terrified to see him in the room with so many cords hooked up to him. *Wet hands. Cord.* A nurse, a doctor, a social worker, so many people asked me to recount what had happened. I began to explain, and Emi jumped in to tell them, "Mommy can tell you her version of the story, and then *I'll* tell you what *really* happened." The suspicion that fell upon me in that moment was a thing I could feel, the sound of mental accusations being leveled, the weight of reports being filed.

But I noticed everyone relax as I hugged Emi tight and told her of course she could tell her version of what happened, she might have seen different things than the things I saw, and that the grown-ups needed to hear both versions, the grown-up Mommy one and the big-sister one. She sat with coloring books and graham crackers and juice while I choked out the version of events as I understood them, still hyperventilating through tears of shock and guilt.

What I told them: That as far as I could tell, from what I had been able to make sense of, he had left the bathroom with his hands still slightly damp from washing, and had reached under the couch to get his car. In doing so, he had touched an extension cord where one of the plugs was not fully flush with the socket. He suffered an electrical shock and passed out and went into seizures.

What I did not tell them: The plug upon which he seized was the plug that powered my laptop. My computer. My work. The instrument I used to write about them, my children. The thing that simultaneously enabled me to be proximal to them while also taking me away from them, enabling me to be in the room with them, perhaps even writing something about them, some anecdote or story, while utterly being absent from them outside of a *Hmmm?* or a *Sure, that sounds like fun* in response to who even knows what was being said.

What I told them: I hadn't seen it happen, I was still in the bathroom. I'd just heard it happen, and then ran as soon as I could.

What I did not tell them: I was in the bathroom, looking at myself in the mirror as I put on makeup.

Once they were done, they went to Emi, and I could hear her begin to tell her story of how Nate floated up to the ceiling as he died.

Within hours, he improved. He was able to talk to us again, and while the doctors did their doctoring, I tried to distract him with questions about things we'd done that morning, and he remembered them, so I was hopeful. He perked up a bit more and then wanted to take a nap. I was terrified to see him sleep, but the doctors said it should be fine. I stayed with him at the hospital for as long as I could, then Gil took over and I went home to be with Emi, who was still shaken, like me, who didn't want to sit near the couch where he had faded away, who was upset that she had ripped her Belle costume dress and demanded that I sew it right then with my shaking hands on the couch where I thought Nate had died, who was worried that maybe she might have made Nate die a little because she wished he was dead sometimes. She couldn't get the pictures out of her head, she told me, so she started to draw them. Page after page of Nate looking dead, or floating, his eyes rolled back in his head, little panic lines to indicate him shaking from a seizure.

The next morning, at the hospital, it was as if Nate was supercharged. When he saw me, he lit up and gave me a big hug and kiss, and when I said, "Oh, Nate, you're so sweet!" he replied, "Oh, Mommy! That's just love!"

"I was so worried about you," I told him, and he said, "But Mommy, I was so worried about you, too! And you know what? I just love you, all the time. I'm just always going to love you!"

He was fine, but I was not. Because I'd thought all of that was gone. When he was lying there on the couch seizing and turning blue, I thought all of that—all of that personality, the sweet brilliance of a kid who could happily and freely reassure me that he was just always going to love me—I'd thought that was gone forever. And even once I knew it wasn't, I was still somehow perpetually stuck in that awful moment when I was on the phone with 911 and he was dying and I was so sure that my own death was the only way I would be able to survive it.

He was fine, but Emi and I were not. I tried to cope by staying in motion, so as to keep at bay the impulse of my mind to replay those endless scenes of my running around the corner, finding him slumped against the wall, his face turning lifeless and gray. In every small moment of rest, I would relive it, and so I tried to remain restless, doing what I could to keep the flood at bay. Emi coped by allowing the flood. "Let's talk about how Nate died," she would say, while coloring or getting ready for bed, and this was the last thing I wanted to talk about, the thing I was endlessly trying to prevent my mind from chattering at me about. And yet I knew this was her way of processing, to create a narrative to understand the trauma, and thus tame it. I suggested, "How about we think of it like a book, a very long book that we can't read all at once because it's just too long to read at bedtime, and we read a chapter at a time together and then put it away?" And she agreed. And so each night, we'd lie there in the dark, and she'd narrate the story of how Nate died but didn't die, and I would will my body to be calm next to her, embracing her, even as my heart hammered in my chest and every nerve ending I had seemed to scream *He's dead, he's dead, you have killed him.*

The first weekend after the accident, Emi requested a "Mommy-Emi" weekend, so that we could spend time together, just us. I wasn't sure whether this was a good idea, for us to be alone—after all, we had experienced Nate's accident alone, just the two of us. And yet her impulse to create a different, more positive bonding experience for us was a good one. Gil took Nate to his parents, and Emi made a list of all the things she thought we should do: bubble baths, s'mores, going to the shoe store to look for fancy shoes, going to a "grown-up" yoga class, playing dress-up, doing art projects, playing beauty parlor, watching movies and eating popcorn, sleeping in my bed together. I marveled at her natural impulse toward healing, this restorative, remarkable combination of ordinary and extraordinary things.

It was a good weekend for both of us. At the yoga class, which she managed to keep up with, and which I managed to survive without a panic attack during the quiet moments, she accepted the compliments of the teacher with grace, and when a fellow class-goer we knew asked her "How is your little brother?"—unaware of what had happened, or what a loaded question that might be—Emi responded, "He's fine, thanks," with a smile. But these things, too, were fragile: On the way home from the shoe-shopping portion of our weekend together, she tripped and fell, ripping her tights and skinning her knee, and I sat with her on the sidewalk, crying along with her as she sobbed and shook in my arms, the grief of everything finally pouring out.

The further we moved away from the event, the more things shifted in my memory, in much the same way Emi's narrative changed and shifted as she retold it to me and to others. Lying in bed together in the dark those nights as she read a chapter at a time from the Big Book of Nate Almost Dying, it wasn't that she was lying or confabulating; it really *felt* to her as though she saw sparks shoot out of Nate's body, it really *felt* to her as though she saw a lightning bolt descend from the ceiling and cause him to fade away, even though of course he never dissolved into thin air; even though, like me, she never saw the actual incident, only the second or so afterward. I couldn't argue with the validity of her interpretations. I couldn't say that any of it wasn't true. What about me and my own memory? What is more important or true, the memory of clumsily stabbing at the phone, trying and failing to dial 911? The memory of realizing he was gray and not breathing? Is it true that his heart stopped for a moment, that after he stopped seizing and stopped breathing he really truly was dead? Or is that only how it felt to me? I'd had an eyeliner pencil in my hand when I ran out of the bathroom to find him. I must have still held it when I'd picked him up off the floor and put him on the couch. Days later I found it lodged between the couch cushions, an indictment of my narcissism, my own self-involvement. And yet when I encountered it, I almost couldn't recognize it for what it was—was this one of Emi's pencils? How did this get here? Who put it there? It seemed so out of place. I'd completely forgotten that I'd been holding it when the accident happened. But there it was, reminding me that not everything I remembered was true, and that maybe some things I remembered weren't.

It took maybe a year to be able to stop living in the parallel world of what might have been, to stop being suspended in that limbo where it was eternally Monday and I was on the phone with 911 and Nate was dying. Every day I had proof that he was fine, that the only actual consequence of the accident was my own inability to shake the shadow of the event itself. I couldn't write; I stopped writing about my children; even just using that laptop made me sick to my stomach, despite the fact that I knew I was not literally killing them by typing out an anecdote. It took time, and then a serious deadline, to get me out of that guilty funk. *Deadline.* Eventually I bought a new laptop, a new extension cord, and got back to work.

Would I have actually killed myself if Nate had died? I had been berating myself for my selfishness—for writing about my children; for using a tool to write about my children that had, due to the poor placement of its power cord, nearly killed one of them; for the narcissism of looking at myself in the mirror putting makeup on; for the narcissism of writing down stories to make my life more interesting—and yet how incredibly selfish was the thought of killing myself? To make it even worse, to scale the absolute heights of selfishness, I'd had that thought literally as my other child was in front of me, terrified, more in need of me in that moment than ever. And yet that was my thinking. How could I even consider it, even in a moment of desperation? If he was dead, and then I killed myself, she would have two people to mourn, her six-year-old mind would not be coping with pictures and restorative weekend plans, she would be traumatized for life. And yet that is the thought I felt more certain about than any other thought that day, the memory that haunts me more than almost any other part of that series of events that replayed itself in my mind like the sickest movie: That I would die, too, and that I would deserve it.

But no one died. Not Nate, and not me. Instead I watched them both heal. I marveled at their natural tendencies toward health, at their natural impulses toward recovery. "Trauma doesn't have to be traumatic," my therapist told me, and I watched that statement unfold as a true life experience. Nate had no memory of the accident, no lingering effects from it, and although he was aware of the attention and anxiety of the adults around him, he moved on from it even better than could have been expected. And Emi prescribed herself art therapy, suggested healing activities and rituals, stunned me with her innate sense of resiliency and emotional integrity. They could do this at six and three.

Even my foggy brain is capable of thinking: *How could I even think of asking them to do this at fifteen and twelve?* I already see them struggling to cope, Nate's natural buoyant happiness giving way to anxiety, Emi freezing, unable to turn her stress into art just yet.

Mirror-me at the medicine cabinet tallying up my medications, plotting my way out, is for a moment indistinguishable from the mirror-me of almost a decade ago, putting on eyeliner and dreading the endless task of filling up the hours until bedtime, calculating the odds of whether at least one kid will take a nap so she can work on an article, or write a quick draft, or just have a fucking break, one moment to herself before she has to cut up more fruit and make who knows what for dinner and sew a Belle costume and settle another fight and read two sets of stories and wait in the dark for the tiny voices of children to quiet down into the breath of children on the edge of sleep until she can finally go work on something or sleep herself. Mirror-me at the medicine cabinet sees the mirror-me before the accident, completely oblivious to what will happen next, no idea that the eyeliner in her hand is an accusation, no idea that her dread of the quotidian is a thing she will regret, will pray for in the adrenaline-sick moments ahead of her, will swear to never again take for granted, although of course she will, we all do, eventually, as we forget and become impatient with everything all over again. Mirror-me at the medicine cabinet and mirror-me before the accident merge into one me for a moment and the small buried part of my brain that is still me says *No, this is not a viable plan, no matter how much proof you have that they will be okay, that they have it in them, both of them, to thrive and to survive trauma. No, they will not find you, they will not dial *11 and 811 and 711 before finally dialing 911 and screaming for someone to hurry, they will not promise themselves that if you are really dead, they will kill themselves, they will not be trapped in that moment forever, wishing they, too, were dead.*

And of course my brain agrees with this.

This is what my brain does now: It agrees with itself. And so I find myself thinking *Of course. These medicines are not a plan. I will not take them all at once. I will throw them out at some point. Good idea! Good thinking!*

I go back to bed. My friend has texted again.

"Didn't mean to minimize," it says.

"No problem!" I respond. "Going to sleep now."

"You'll probably feel better after a nap."

I won't. But I recognize that's just his brain trying to be agreeable too. I push all the pillows aside to be as flat as possible, to make the pain as small as possible, put on a podcast, and float in the fog of Britain and the run-up to World War I. I hear the interviewer talking to a group of historians about the deaths of so many young people, and eventually I fall asleep.

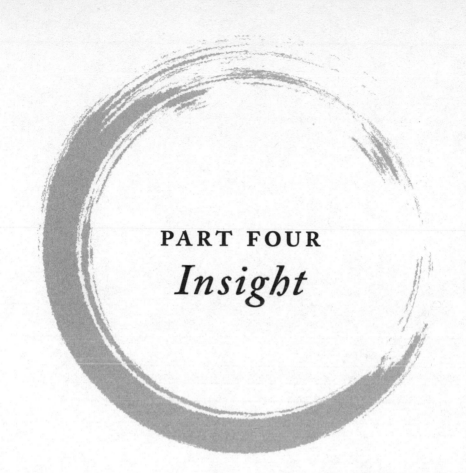

PART FOUR
Insight

The prototypical manifestation of spontaneous intracranial hypotension is an orthostatic headache. Such a headache generally occurs or worsens within 15 minutes of assuming the upright position . . . but in some patients this lag period may be as long as several hours. Improvement of the headache after lying down is less variable and occurs within 15 to 30 minutes. The headache may be diffuse or localized to the frontal, temporal, or—most commonly—the occipital or suboccipital regions. The headache may be throbbing or nonthrobbing and is rarely unilateral. Some patients use descriptive terms for their headaches, such as the feeling of "an ice cube in an empty glass" or a "pulling sensation from my head down to my neck," offering a clue to the diagnosis. Additional clues may be the patient's recumbent position in the physician's office or a pillow they carry along to allow them to lie down comfortably . . . . The severity of the headache varies widely; many mild cases probably remain undiagnosed, whereas other patients are incapacitated and unable to engage in any useful activity while upright.

—Wouter I. Schievink, "Spontaneous Spinal Cerebrospinal
Fluid Leaks and Intracranial Hypotension," *JAMA*, 2006

18

September 2015

I have exhausted the resources available to me at the hospital, with its one doctor familiar with CSF leaks and its many specialists who are not, and so I make an appointment to be seen at a different hospital, one with a headache center and neurologists who specialize in headaches of all kinds. I'm still toying with the idea of trying to reach out to the doctor of last resort, the specialist I've read about online, but my case seems too pedestrian, despite the way it's taken over my life. It just doesn't seem serious enough to merit a cross-country trip, my scans not dramatic enough, my symptoms not definitive enough. Although I don't know what the threshold is, I'm sure I haven't cleared it. And so this is the next step I feel I can take: to be seen by the headache center.

Before I can be evaluated by the headache center, I must go through a screening process. First I am required to take the Minnesota Multiphasic Personality Inventory test, which costs $300, will not be covered by insurance, and takes about an hour to ninety minutes to complete. Then I must meet with one of the headache center's therapists, even though I already have a therapist. But I've run out of other options, so fine: I will take the expensive test, I will talk to the random therapist.

The center itself, which is less a center than a nondescript area on the second floor of the neurology building, presents as a fluorescent-lit waiting room with no place to lie down, which is how I evaluate everything at this point: *Is it dark? Is there a place for me to be flat?* It's taken me more than a half-hour of being upright to get here, and so I am woozy with pain and brain fog, but I nod my head as the desk person informs me that insurance probably won't reimburse me for the cost of the personality test and I sign a thing and take a sheaf of forms to a chair in the corner that seems like the least obnoxious place to lie on the floor if I have to.

The personality inventory test I have to take, the MMPI, is "the most widely used and widely researched objective measure of psychopathology in history," according to what I read about it later, and was first developed in the 1930s. It was initially used to diagnose hypochondriasis, depression, hysteria, psychopathic deviate, paranoia, psychasthenia (an outdated term for what is now considered obsessive-compulsive disorder), schizophrenia, and hypomania. Later, social introversion and masculinity-femininity (measuring how rigidly a person conforms to stereotypical gender roles) were added, creating ten basic diagnostic categories. Beginning in the 1980s, the test underwent a major overhaul, and by

2003, the MMPI-2 was introduced, with clinical scales intended to measure the perhaps more modern states of demoralization, somatic complaints, low positive emotions, cynicism, antisocial behavior, ideas of persecution, dysfunctional negative emotions, aberrant experiences, and hypomanic activation.

The test consists of 567 true/false questions. Some of them are innocuous and easy to answer, though in some cases oddly specific: "I wake up fresh and rested most mornings." "I like mechanics magazines." "I am very seldom troubled by constipation."

Others are clearly red flags: "I am sure I get a raw deal from life." "Evil spirits possess me at times." "I see things or animals or people around me that others do not see." "If people had not had it in for me I would have been much more successful."

But others are harder to answer: "There seems to be a lump in my throat much of the time." "No one seems to understand me." "I have nightmares every few nights." "I have had very peculiar and strange experiences." "Much of the time my head seems to hurt all over." "I get angry sometimes." "I wish I could be as happy as others seem to be."

Those seem like traps, those seem as though answering truthfully—yes, my head *does* hurt all over pretty much all the time, I really *have* had strange experiences, this entire *thing* is a strange experience, I *do* get angry about it sometimes, I *do* wish I were happy like people who aren't in pain all the time—would result in a therapist thinking, *Uh-oh.* And after reading through all these questions, I'm halfway beginning to believe the more obviously troubling ones that suggest a conspiracy may be afoot—A surprise brain leak, of all things? Constant pain? A divorce? Maybe the world really *is* out to get me! Maybe this *is* a message from the universe that I am a bad person! Maybe this *is* some kind of plot!

But I do my best to answer the questions, asking myself, *How would a normal person answer these questions, how would*

I answer these questions if my head weren't hurting all the time and my brain worked the way it was supposed to?—even though I suspect the test may be designed to take into account people who try to take it thinking *How would a normal person answer these questions?*

By the time I finish the questionnaire, I have more than surpassed my limit for sitting up, and the scrapey feeling that feels like my brain chafing and grating against my skull—*even though it can't actually be that feeling*, I remind myself, my fingers massaging the back of my head anyway, as if I could launch my brain away from the hard edge of my skull like an inflatable toy floating across a swimming pool—is unbearable. But before I can speak with the neurologists, I must meet with one of the center's in-house therapists. I'm escorted to her blessedly dark office, everything muted and somber out of respect for the migraine patients, and I gamely attempt to answer her questions as I slide farther and farther down the chair, trying to be flat. Eventually, I lie on the floor. Yes, I've had a constant headache for six months at this point. Yes, I've been told this is due to a spontaneous CSF leak. Sure, I can define what a CSF leak is. Yes, it has been stressful. Yes, I am in the midst of a divorce. Yes, I have a therapist I see regularly. Yes, my headache affects my quality of life. Yes, I spend most of the day flat, in bed, because gravity is a thing, and when I stand up, I lose more fluid around my brain. Yes, I have tried various treatments for the CSF leak. No, they have not worked.

After listening to me speak for a while, the therapist tells me about some yoga and meditation classes the center offers, some biofeedback programs. I nod and comment that right now it's hard for me to get anywhere or do anything that involves being upright. "I hear that," she tells me. "In fact, it seems like you are pretty alone and isolated right now. We've got to get you out of bed and socializing! Seeing friends! Interacting!" I remind her, through tears, the reason I am here, lying on the floor of her office, is because I literally can't sit up. That I am at level nine pain on their dumb ten-point pain scale all the time, even when I'm flat. That "socializing" is an impossible luxury for me. That I'm being seen at the headache center to have my CSF leak evaluated, to hopefully get it repaired. Not because I'm lonely. "Ah," she says. "Right." Session over!

While I wait for the neurologists, I fill out yet another form, a headache questionnaire I will be asked to fill out every time I have an appointment. It takes a few months of visits for me to realize that this is busywork, that they never actually look over what I've written down, despite how much I agonize over getting it right.

> Are there any events that have affected your headache?
> _____Yes _____No

There is an inch-long line to describe these possible events. I circle *Yes* and write as small as I can: "I developed a spontaneous CSF leak in March 2015."

> Frequency: Number of headache days weekly _____
> Number of headache days monthly _____

This is nearly impossible to answer. I don't have headaches, I have *headache*. One long, ever-lasting permanent headache. I write "7" for the number of days a week I have a headache. For the number of headache days monthly, I write, "All the days."

> Have you had any headache-free periods?
> _____Yes _____No. If yes, _____hours _____all day

The mere concept of headache-free periods confuses me. I can't imagine minutes without a headache, let alone hours. The suggestion of a headache-free time that lasts all day seems particularly cruel. I circle *No*.

On a scale of 0–10, how severe are your headaches?
____/10 Mild ones ____/10 Severe ones ____/10 Average ones

This, too, is hard to answer. There is no difference in the amount of pain I have, not really. When I lie down, I feel better, but the pain isn't exactly less, it's just different, perhaps less unrelenting maybe. Pain is a slippery thing. I've had two children, I've had a kidney stone, I've thrown my back out, I've had a toothache, I've had paper cuts, I've had blistering sunburns, I've had shin splints, I've had my heart broken, I've stepped on a Lego—I've experienced a spectrum of pain, and I know that in the moment of it, pain doesn't feel like something quantifiable, it just feels like pain. When I try to remember the acute pain I've experienced, like for instance with the kidney stone, I remember in an academic sense the agony, the pain so bad I couldn't stop vomiting, the intensity. But what I remember bodily, what I have a clearer, more visceral memory of, is the moment that the stone passed and, unbelievably, I no longer hurt. Lying there on a gurney in the emergency room and suddenly feeling the absence of pain was a legitimate moment of ecstasy, a literal rush of relief, and that's what I remember now, so many years later, more than anything else: the ecstatic pleasure of no longer hurting. Is this pain that bad? If it suddenly stopped, would I yell out "Oh my god, it doesn't hurt anymore!" like I did then? I write in "7" for mild, "9" for severe, "8" for average. I've got to give myself someplace to go, I reason. Maybe this could get worse, maybe this isn't a 10 yet. But I don't know.

Have your headache symptoms or location changed?
_____ Yes _____ No

This is also difficult to answer. Since the blood patch a few months ago, things have changed. Instead of the pain mostly being centered on the right side, it's sometimes on the left now, too; and I have the scrapey-head headache now, that's new. And of course right after the blood patch, I spent weeks feeling as though my head was about to explode, that was a change in symptoms. Too much pressure instead of not enough, like the worst cold or sinus infection, my head as tight as a balloon, ready to pop. But were those symptoms, really? That all seems like a reaction to the blood patch procedure rather than something new, or something diagnostically meaningful. I circle *Yes* and write in: "Changes in location and quality since blood patch."

Are you able to work?
_____ Yes _____ No. If no, please explain why

There is another inch-long line for the explanation. I stare at this question for a while. I circle *No*, obviously, but I'm at a loss as to what I can possibly say to explain my answer. It seems like it should be self-evident. It feels humiliating to have to answer. I feel anxious even acknowledging the question. Finally, I write: "Because I can't think." I don't really know what else to say.

When I meet with the neurologist, all the prescreen hurdles conquered, I hand her the questionnaire and she tucks it away with other papers on her desk. I tell her my history: the flu, the cough, the MRIs, the attempts at bed rest and medication, the CT scan that showed I had a broken neck that has nothing to do with the leak, the way the doctors thought the leak might be somewhere in my ethmoid sinus but maybe not, the canceled through-the-face surgery with the ENT, the barbaric blood patch; the way my head threatened to explode after, the way I had more upright time after, the way I was able to do a little bit more but still felt so foggy, still felt so much pain, still got worse as the day went on, still couldn't be upright for too long at a time. I tell her about the pain, about the drunk feeling, the way it feels like the thinking part of my brain is turned off and I'm just on autopilot, talking too much, just like when I'm tipsy, moving and speaking without thinking; the way it feels as though the part of my brain that's in charge is the part that can ramble, fake, simulate, literally go through the motions. She listens to me and calls in another neurologist, and I go over it all again as they look at my chart, scan the question-naire, thumb through my records.

What they tell me is that it sounds like I am definitely still leaking. That the blood patch might have helped, but not enough, because it wasn't high enough on my spine, and so it can only do so much to create a kind of temporary roadblock, a constricting place that forces the cerebrospinal fluid upward a little bit. These neurologists aren't confused by my symptoms; the recitation of my history isn't met with immediate skepticism and doubt. They have encountered spinal CSF leaks before in their practice, and have experience in treating at least the symptoms. They recommend another round of MRIs; a round of steroids; a series of infusion treatments, a bolus of fluids and pain medications to bust through that secondary brain-scraping headache; if neces-sary, another blood patch. "But can you *fix* the leak?" I ask, and they say they can't. They don't know where it is, and even if they had the diagnostic machines and experience to find it, they still wouldn't be able to patch it shut. They don't have doctors here with the training to be able to do that. There are places that do, out-of-state hospitals I could travel to if necessary. "But this is the next step," they tell me. "It's still possible for the leak to resolve itself, and these treatments will offer some relief while we wait and see if that happens."

Wait and see, wait and see, always more waiting and seeing. The waiting seems impossible. But it feels good, a little bit, to be seen.

19

October 2015

M ore MRIs showing nothing. More CT scans showing nothing. I remember when I felt relieved, at first, that there was nothing, that no one was calling to tell me the scans had bloomed with tumors flowering throughout my brain. But now, after so many months, my unremarkable brain scans feel accusatory. Almost taunting. I haven't read the literature at this point, I don't know that it is common for someone with a spinal CSF leak to have nothing show up on an MRI, and so my non-results feel like yet more evidence pointing to this whole thing as mere malingering. Perhaps this is all imagined, this pain. Perhaps I feel compelled to seek out attention from doctors because I am divorcing a doctor.

This is ridiculous, of course: but it's what I imagine my medical notes must look like at this point. Indictments.

I'm on a course of dexamethasone steroids, and mostly what they're doing is keeping my thoughts in motion. I now have impulse, energy, but still no clear brain to execute my plans. I feel compelled to organize, as though the part of me that can still kind of think is seeking out ways to control this, and this translates to me as ideas like *clean out the closet, find a better system for the recycling, fix the squeaky table, gather up those cords, put things in order, make everything clean and understandable,* even if it hurts my head to be upright and doing things. Which makes sense because everything is such a fog, everything is floating away from me as I lie in bed after organizing things, my head aching, even as the steroids course through me. I listen to podcasts and play Tetris-like games on my phone, fitting things neatly into other things, puzzling things into place until there's no more room to fit them. It's satisfying because right now nothing's fitting, or perhaps because so many things are flitting away from me. And so it gives me a feeling of purpose, to do things, even if I'm doing them on autopilot: *get the plate, put food on plate, bring to table, clear away, place in sink, fold laundry, put laundry away.* The pleasure of things where they belong.

It's helpful, this impulse to do things, but it's also dangerous, because I can't properly evaluate whether or not any of the things I'm doing are worthwhile. Some of them are, of course—making dinner for the kids, being guided through the steps as if I'm a vessel receiving instructions from beyond—but maybe if I were fully me, my brain fully working right now, I'd be realizing *No, that's not a good idea, order pizza, don't stand up and waste time draining more of your precious brain fluid away.* Or I'd be making lists of things I'd like to organize and clean and accomplish once I'm feeling better instead of just going along with this primal organizing brain and doing things I don't really have to do. I go to the paint store and buy paint and paint a bathroom. I spackle the holes in the wall where the towel rack fell out, and I sand the spackled place, and I tape up the molding, and I paint with bright blue paint, and I climb on a ladder, and I get tiny blue spray dots on the ceiling, and in between all of these things I lie down on the floor, listening to podcasts and waiting for my brain fluid to regenerate a bit before I get up and keep going. I go back to the paint store and get more paint and start painting a wall in the basement. The steroids keep me going, but I know it's not a good idea, that every second I stand up, my cerebrospinal fluid is draining away, my headache increasing. And yet I paint until the small bucket of paint runs out. I lie down on the floor and decide it's fine to leave the wall unfinished. It's not even a major wall, not a wall someone would even see if they walked downstairs into the basement. If they happened to go to the basement and turn a corner and then look to the right, they'd see it. But it's not like it matters. This makes sense to me. This project is done for now. I can finish it later, when I'm healed.

Am I ever going to be healed?

I'm worried I'm going to be trapped here forever. I'm worried this will never go away, that I will always be leaking. How messy of me, how clumsy, how gauche, to be leaking, uncontained, how undignified. I'm worried if it does go away, it will happen again and again. I'm worried I may never fully recover from this. I'm worried about it lasting so long that my symptoms become permanent, even if I do manage to get healed.

This worry isn't anything that can be seen on an MRI. But that doesn't mean it's not there.

The steroids are helping me power through this, but I can still feel everything slipping away. And what happens when this course of medication is over? Will I be debilitated like before? Will my headache return to being unbearable, will my hands disappear, will I be back to being in a permanent state of confusion? The steroids are giving me the imperative to Do Things, but I know how this works. This, too, will slip away, and then it'll be back to bed, staring at the ceiling, listening to podcasts, tethering myself to the sound of conversations even if I can't really follow what's being said.

I can't stay like this. I need this to be fixed. It's taking so long. I'm worried it won't be fixed. The doctors here can't fix me, they can only give me steroids, pain medicine, blood patches. I'm afraid of having another blood patch, straight-up terrified. And I'm worried that it will fail once again.

Who am I if I can't think like me? Who will I become if I keep thinking like this?

20

I am an unreliable narrator.

My children bear the burden of my flawed storytelling.

Is the story I've been telling them about this divorce, the time-line, the breakdown, the true one? No. But it is the story they can bear. And the story of my brain, of what's happening to me, of this leak: I don't know enough to tell them the true story, the full story. I can only flesh out what they already know: that I'm in pain, that I am unavailable to them in a way I haven't been before. That I look like me, but I am a poor facsimile of myself. My imagined story of what their story of me is now is one of anger and betrayal. How dare I become a ghost, how dare I haunt them from this body that looks like their mother but has somehow given up on being their mother, at the same time their father has given up on being their father. They do not tell me this story. But over and over again, I imagine it.

How fitting a metaphor, this losing of my mind; how else must it appear to them? Of course their mother has lost her mind. What other explanation could there be for suddenly abandoning this marriage, abandoning the stability of their lives? Of course their mother's brain is struggling to function, the mother they knew slowly leaking away, a bathtub draining, a blown-up raft deflating. That is the only way this could be happening. What other explanation could be possible? That I would *choose* this?

And in their story, if I become fixed, does that fix them, too? There could be a version of this story in which instead of this family leaking away, becoming smaller, it comes together, it rallies, their dad sticks by me, we stay together. They don't understand that this part of the story has been foretold, that developments have taken place in a prequel they haven't read. The only way this comes together is by breaking apart, reconfiguring. But they can't see that. They see me flat, or standing, confused, my illness becoming a part of the general parental drone. *Lights off, take a shower, get your shoes on, brush your teeth, eat your food before it gets cold, take a sweater, my head is killing me.* I worry this is killing them.

Back in the fog again, I'm rendered incapable of narrative. And yet once I'm there, flat, in the fog, the me who is Me safely tucked away in a fortress of pain, reduced to merely acknowledging that thoughts exist, I can see how clearly my thoughts behave without me to direct them. This, I will remember later, is the aim of all the books I have read on Buddhism, all the meditation podcasts I have listened to, all the teachings I've encountered: to understand that you are not your thoughts, and your thoughts are not you.

But this doesn't feel like enlightenment, as I struggle to think, as I sense a part of my brain continuing on without me. It feels terrifying.

The Buddhists have a word for that, too: *groundlessness.*

Enveloped in fog, I'm faced with the limits of my storytelling, the fruitlessness of storytelling.

Attempting to trace this back to the beginning of everything is merely an exercise. Coming up with a theory, a plausible fairy tale, of how it started doesn't change the facts of where I am now. Telling myself the story of how my relationship unraveled doesn't knit it back together. Following the trail back into the past changes nothing about the present.

And yet this is the work of the self. This is the work of the brain, the work of the mind: creating narrative, finding patterns, puzzling things into place.

This is the work I must do with my children: help them understand the story of their lives, help them place these things in a context, help them frame a narrative around the disruption of everything they've known.

And yet don't these stories just distract? Don't they obfuscate? Don't they hide the truth, which is that there is no narrative, and nothing makes sense, and there is no pattern, and the world is uncaring, cruel, no lessons to learn, no moral, no upside, just the brutal facts of this happening, and then this happening, and then this happening?

I tell them: There are lots of different ways to be a family. I tell them: Look at all the people you know in your life and the way their families are, the way your friends seamlessly move between one household and another, the way it is just a fact that they have two families, or two moms, or two dads, or four moms, or three places to go. These people are on the other side of where you are, but at one point they were here, where you are now, confused and upset and unsure about how to navigate this transition. There is a map for this, and while someone else's map won't look exactly like yours, and the terrain you travel to get where you're going might be different from theirs, it is a path you can follow. This is a thing other people have done. Our family isn't the first to change its configuration.

I tell them: Here are the things that won't change—that I love you, and that you will always come first in my heart; that your dad loves you, and that he always will, no matter whether he lives here or somewhere else. I tell them: This isn't the ending of the story, although it feels like the end. This is somewhere in the middle, a turning point, a journey into the woods where a protagonist wanders, seemingly alone, and encounters magical, secret things that will change them profoundly. It's the part where things seem bleakest. The part before the part where everything turns out fine.

I tell them stories, I tell them to think of stories, even though I doubt the power of stories to do anything but lie about the painful truth of this pain, physical, emotional, that affects us all.

In fact, we have all been betrayed by the story I've been telling.

The story I've been telling them—that everything is okay, that the way things are in our house is normal, sustainable—is a lie. The story I've been telling them about our lives—that everything is stable and dependable, that feelings pass and that brains are powerful and that reframing things to better understand them is the right way to cope—is a lie. The true story is that things are not fine, that things are not sustainable, that things are out of our control, that pain cannot be mitigated, that making things work means acknowledging that they are broken, unfixable. But how can I tell them that?

I have been a storyteller like the narrators in fairy tales, beginning and ending things with the hand-wavey vagueness of once upon a times and happily ever afters. I have been a storyteller of bright sides and best-case scenarios, a storyteller whose narrative job has been to make it easy for my listeners to believe that everything's okay, that everything ends well, that they are safe. As a storyteller, I should have better warned them of, should have better foreshadowed, the surprise of things falling apart.

I wanted to give them a story of continuity, predictability, dependability, so they could trust, be secure, not be seduced by the anxiety of intermittent reinforcement. And so it seems doubly cruel to reveal to them the plot twist that nothing is as it seems, that their mostly placid home life is a frozen surface with angry currents churning beneath, that their dependable, omnipresent mother is actually absent, restricted, distant, lost to them in the confines of her bed, that everything they thought they knew is actually just a story, and the story is a lie.

And so it is true: I am an unreliable narrator.

In telling them this story—of my illness, of the divorce—I should be calm, calculated, completely in control of the telling, so that it sounds to them like a story about a runaway rock turning into a landslide and everyone making it out alive, instead of the story itself becoming a runaway rock turning into a landslide, with no guarantees of survival. I should make them feel confident that they are in good hands, that I'm trustworthy and above emotion, not part of the audience experiencing it, or held captive to it. And yet I am not in control of this story. I am beyond narrative; I am unable to frame these events in a way that feels safe and makes sense. I am tumbling down the mountain with them, instead of telling them a story of what it's like to tumble down the mountain.

And yet the only way I can see our way through it is with more stories. So I try my best, I continue my unreliable narration. Here is the story of how our lives will be different: weekend schedules and taking turns, custody and visiting hours. Here is the story of how our lives will stay the same: home is home, and school is school, and love is love, that doesn't change. Here is the story of how we grow apart and grow back together; here is the story of how we become a different kind of family; here is the story of remarriage and recon-figuration and reforming and reemergence. Here is the story of how we move forward when I am stuck in time, my brain compromised, my pain constant, as aching and omnipresent as their emotional pain, my existential trauma as traumatic as theirs. Here is the plan for how we will do this, slowly and step by step, walking through the fog, limited by how little we can see before us. Here is how we get through this. Here are the stories we will tell ourselves.

It seems cruel and pointless and not enough, but stories are all we have.

21

October 2015

My sister Jessie drives me to the hospital for my second blood patch. I lie down in the car, I lie down in the waiting room, wedged sideways in a double-wide chair. I lie down everywhere. She's allowed to come with me as I'm escorted to a room, a curtained-off area with a bed and a rolling side table and a television tuned to a *Law & Order* marathon. I change into the starchy hospital gown, the fuzzy socks with nubs on the bottom to keep me from slipping in case of some fleeting moment when I might be upright, and lie on the bed, blissfully flat. A nurse comes in and asks me a few questions, including one I find slightly odd: "How long ago did you give birth?" I raise an eyebrow and say, "I mean,

142

the last time was roughly 13 years ago?" and we both laugh an uncomfortable laugh, and we are both confused as to which one of us might be joking. "You *are* here for a blood patch, right?" she asks, and I say yes, and then she leaves, and my sister and I look at each other like *What was that about?*

We watch television and make small talk while we wait; Jessie checks in with her boss on the phone, I lie flat and doze off and on. My procedure is scheduled for 10 A.M., but soon it is 10:30, 11, 11:30, and no one is coming for me. Jessie has heard the stories about my experiences with hospitals and this leak, with the last blood patch I had, the mix-ups and delays and confusion; she jokes that this must be par for the course, just the way these things seem to go for me, but pushes aside the curtain to go find the nurse in charge of things and discover what's causing the delay.

After some discussion, my sister returns, followed by the nurse, who apologizes and tells me she's actually been on the phone for the past 45 minutes, trying to figure out what's going on. It appears that the neurology fellow who scheduled this procedure has arranged for me to be in the wrong department of the hospital. I'm currently in the place where women who have recently given birth are treated for post-dural puncture headaches—CSF leaks due to faulty administration of epidural anesthesia. These women are given epidural blood patches the way my first one was done, sitting up, leaning on a resident or nurse while an anesthesiologist shoots them blindly with blood in the same spot where some other anesthesiologist's needle pierced their dura. The part of the hospital where I was supposed to be scheduled is the chronic pain center, in the neuroscience building—the place where anesthesiologists work in operating rooms, where they can give patients oxygen and pain relief and perform blood patches using fluoroscopy, which I now know is a kind of X-ray imaging, giving them a better view of what they're doing, and cutting down on the chance of piercing the dura yet again and causing a new leak. Because my neurologist scheduled me at this place instead of that one, the anesthesiology team that should be performing my procedure is booked for the day, and so it seems I will not be having a blood patch after all. "I'm sorry," the nurse says, "I know you're in a lot of pain. Has this been going on for a while?" I start to cry from sheer frustration as I tell her, "Almost seven months, I can't take it anymore," and I see her frown in determination, and something changes in her, and she squeezes my hand and tells me to sit tight.

My sister says, "Wow, you really weren't kidding about this stuff being ridiculous. What is this, your second day of being in a hospital for a thing you don't actually get to have done?", and I text Gil to let him know what's going on. Things are tense between us of course, due to the ongoing and seemingly everlasting negotiations over our divorce, but we are united in agreement on a few things: one, the importance of making things as easy as possible throughout this process for our kids, and two, his natural strength in advocating and arguing with fellow medical professionals. So I text him, and he calls me, and I tearfully explain today's clusterfuck, and he kicks into gear, making phone calls and going what the kids and I affectionately refer to as "full Binenbaum" on the doctors involved in what's not happening today. He harangues the neurology fellow to the point where I almost feel bad for her as she calls me to apologize for the mix-up, sounding close to tears herself, and he chops through a phone tree until he finally reaches a person from the pain department who can come see me and help figure out what to do.

The nurse returns, telling me that she, too, has been making phone calls, and has also talked to Gil, and that they are tag-teaming the higher-ups who might be able to fix this and make a blood patch happen today after all, and then a resident from the pain clinic comes in, seeming bored by all of this—my tears, my pain, my frustration, my hours of waiting—and says the best they can do is shunt me over to the doctor's office across the street, where I can be interviewed and my case reviewed, and then they can schedule me for the procedure at some later date. The resident hands me paperwork, and a Post-it note with a phone number on it for the receptionist at the pain clinic, and leaves in a breeze of curtain swishing—but the nurse takes the papers from my hands. "I did not make fifty phone calls on your behalf today to have this happen," she tells me. "You need this done, we're gonna get this done." She tells me she knows the head nurse at the pain clinic, who happens to be working today in the OR where the anesthesiology team is equipped to perform a blood patch, and that she will spend her fifty-first phone call of the day calling this head nurse to work some magic and get me in.

And she does. She makes the call, and while I can't hear enough to know exactly what she is saying, I can hear the righteous anger on my behalf, the frustration and determination in her voice, and it makes me cry all over again to hear her fight for me. And then she is back, discharge papers in hand, telling me to change back into my street clothes, that she will escort me across the street and deliver me in person to the nursing staff at the chronic pain department of the hospital for neuroscience, where the head of anesthesiology himself will fit me in as the last case of the day. My sister helps me fill out the release forms, I lie down after getting dressed until the nurse can take us where we need to go, and then we walk outside, me unsteadily, slowly, supported by the strong arm of the nurse, the sun bright in my eyes after hours inside, and reach the pain center—oh, if only there were a center to my pain, some eye in this storm—by 5 P.M.

"Is this the one you told me about?" the nurse's friend asks. "You poor thing! Let's get this taken care of!" My nurse hugs me and wishes me well as she heads back to the other part of the hospital, hopefully finished with her endless phone calls and patient advocacy on my behalf for the day. I'm quickly ushered to a bed, changed again into the ubiquitous backless gown and skid-free socks, visited by several anesthesiologists and nurses, and asked to go over my history yet again. Everyone is cheerful to me, apologetic, reassuring. The head anesthesiologist says he will attempt to do this blood patch a little higher than my first one, but of course he can't perform the patch too high, even if it might be more effective, because of the risks involved. I understand; I would not like to be paralyzed, even if it might cure my headache. The anesthesiologist explains they will use fluoroscopy to be able to visualize the epidural space in my spine and make sure they are in the right place, able to inject the blood without piercing the dura. They will paint my back with lidocaine, place a catheter in my spine, fill a needle with the blood they collect from me, and push it in. The anesthesiologist examines the backs of my hands, smooth and veinless, and looks longingly at Jessie's hands, snaking blue bulges visible to the naked eye even from his vantage point across the hospital bed. "I've been waiting around since about 9 this morning and haven't anything to drink," I tell him. "It will be impossible to get blood from my hands. What about my arm, inside my elbow?" He considers this, but says they'll be able to do it—if necessary, they can use a vein finder, a special light that illuminates the blood vessels. He disappears and is replaced by a different pain management specialist, who promises me something he calls a fentanyl cocktail during the process. Once they get the IV placed in my hand and extract the blood they need, they'll pump me full of pain relief. This sounds heavenly, so exactly the opposite of my first blood patch experience, that I could cry. "But try not to," my sister says. "You're already so dehydrated."

Soon I am wheeled to an operating room, then rolled over from my back to my stomach onto a table. My head has a pillow placed beneath my chin, my left arm is extended and fitted with a blood pressure cuff, plastic tubing is draped below my nose, vents beneath my nostrils whispering oxygen into my face. My right arm is extended, and a team of gowned and masked medical people peer at the back of my hand, searching in vain for veins. My hand is massaged, squeezed, lightly tapped, lightly slapped, while cold lidocaine is applied low on my spine. "I'm one of those people who needs more lidocaine than normal," I remind the anesthesiologist, and he assures me he'll give me extra and wait a bit longer for it to settle in. "You might have better luck with my arm," I tell the people clustered around my hand, who are now turning the lights low and searching for my veins with the vein finder, but they seem not to be listening to me. The pain management guy who'd promised me the fentanyl cocktail says they can't do it until the IV is placed, and the hand IV is proving quite difficult. The group of doctors managing the IV keep massaging and slapping my hand, while the other half of the group of doctors hovers around my lower back, beginning the process of placing a catheter in my back and injecting me with contrast fluid. This will help them visualize the spinal epidural space as X-rays are continually passed through my body and broadcast to the fluoroscope, a TV-like monitor where they can see a real-time vision of what's going on inside me.

An IV is finally jammed into a vein in my hand, but after several team members consult over it, the vein is deemed unproductive, and so the needle is withdrawn and painfully reinserted in a new spot in my hand. I'm grateful for the oxygen; otherwise I feel I might pass out from the stabbing in my hand, the twinge in my back. The second IV placement isn't much more productive than the first, and two doctors massage and squeeze my hand to make the tapped vein offer up its blood. They need to inject 15 ccs of my own blood into the epidural space in my lower spine—but due to my dehydration and insufficient veins, they're having trouble getting that much. The trick with an epidural blood patch is that the blood needs to be extracted and then injected more or less immediately, before it has a chance to clot. But all they can squeeze out of me is a few ccs at a time, and so they collect 5 ccs and inject it, then wait for 2 more ccs to accumulate and inject that, then wait for a few more ccs to be collected and inject that. This isn't ideal, but they manage to collect and inject and collect and inject and collect and inject something like 11 or 12 ccs total. From my perspective on the table, inhaling oxygen and crying from the pain of my battered hand being milked for blood, it feels like a gradual filling up of my back until I can't tolerate the pressure in my spine anymore, which means that it is over.

But as painful and uncomfortable as it is, lying there on the table, trying not to shiver in the cold dark room, my hand spiked with pain, my other arm squeezed in a cuff, a catheter in my back, and a needle in my spine, for just a moment I experience a revelation. I can actually pinpoint the instant the injection of fluid is enough to bolster my brain and make it float again, because as I lie on the table, I feel myself come back to myself. I find myself exclaiming, through my tears, "Oh my god, I can *think* again," and there is this sudden rush, this undeniable sense of the me who is Me finally emerging from the shadows, fully inhabiting my brain, able to exist again. I hear the head anesthesiologist laugh and say, "Good, it's working," and the pain management guy apologizes for being unable to provide me with that fentanyl cocktail he'd promised and says he'll bring me tramadol, and my back is wiped clean of contrast and medication and blood, and I—me, *Me*, the me who feels like myself, the me who can think—I am turned over onto my side and transferred to a rolling bed on my back and the fluorescent lights move above me and then the tramadol brings me some relief as I lie in the darkened, curtained waiting area, my back sore, my hand purpling from the assault, my brain allowing my mind to feel like myself again.

It takes two weeks for the bruises to fade, so by the time I have my follow-up with the anesthesiologist at the pain clinic, they are yellowish-greenish ghosts on the back of my hand. "How are you feeling?" he asks me, and I tell him I'm not sure. My back and leg didn't feel as bad as they did after the last blood patch—maybe because they did the injection a little higher this time, and also got it in the right space without hitting a nerve—and my head also didn't feel as bad as the last time, no intolerable, head-exploding pressure. But I'm worried, because although I spent at least five days after this blood patch in bed, resting, the fog is back, and the me who is Me is receding again, and the familiar headache is beginning to replace the post–blood patch headache.

"You need to give it some time," he tells me. "With the blood patch, we're compressing the space there so the fluid is pushed upward, but we're also trying to provoke an inflammatory response, so your body will attack the area where the tear is and work to heal it. We need to give it time to do that." I nod my head, even though I know the feeling that I'm feeling is not an inflammatory response, not my brain adjusting to normal pressure, the leak sealed by blood and my body's own insistence, but rather my leak still slowly leaking. The anesthesiologist tells me to keep in touch, reminds me that if I want to try another patch in the next few weeks, I can get in touch with him directly and forget about the neurologists. "We don't need them," he jokes, and I laugh.

Before returning home, I stop off at the floor of the hospital where the nurse works who saved the day for me and got me the blood patch. I hope she's there today: I have brought her a thank-you card, a copy of one of my books. It's all I can think to do, such a small gesture, and I worry on the way that I should have done something better, that maybe instead I should order coffee and donuts for the entire nursing staff of that department, the whole floor.

I feel woozy in the elevator, foggy after being upright for so long getting to my appointment, sitting through my appointment, standing to wait for the elevator. I arrive at the reception area and ask if the nurse is working today, and she is, and I am allowed to go back into the patient area to see her, and she recognizes me and embraces me, and I start to cry as I try to thank her for what she did for me that day, the way she fought for me and took me seriously and shared her fierce compassion. Her hug is strong, and she accepts the gift and my tears, and she says she just hopes I was able to get some relief.

"Did it work?" She asks. "Are you all better now?" I want to be able to tell her yes, that her extraordinary work meant something, helped me find relief, helped me get justice, but she can already see in my eyes the disappointment, the truth. I say, weeping, undermining my own attempt at optimism, "It's too early to tell, really. But I'm standing up now, walking around. You helped me do that." She squeezes my arm and wishes me well and hugs me again. "I hope you get the thing that fixes you," she tells me, and I say, "Me too," and head to the elevators, to a taxi that can take me home.

Large-volume lumbar epidural blood patches, an approach adapted from the treatment of post–lumbar puncture headache, are often used for treatment of spontaneous intracranial hypotension and can be effective immediately. However, it remains unclear how such therapy might actually address the underlying problem of spontaneous CSF leaks, given that when visualized, these leaks are most commonly observed in the thoracic region, not the lumbar region. One possibility is that these nondirected "patches" increase CSF pressure by displacement of volume in the spinal canal, thereby alleviating symptoms until spontaneous closure of leaks can occur. Although this technique can be effective for some patients, it is not as effective as epidural blood patching performed in the setting of post–lumbar puncture headaches, is generally less effective when the patch is placed distant from an identified leak site, and may not achieve durable results in a significant proportion of patients. Reports of the overall rates of success for lumbar epidural blood patching vary significantly. While some series report success rates in excess of 80%, several studies have found success rates to be substantially lower, and several authors have reported success rates of <50%.

—P.G. Kranz, L. Gray, and J.N. Taylor, "CT-Guided Epidural Blood Patching of Directly Observed or Potential Leak Sites for the Targeted Treatment of Spontaneous Intracranial Hypotension," *American Journal of Neuroradiology*, May 2011

22

J ust under two weeks since the second blood patch, it has been determined that the patch has officially failed, and so the next prong of attack is three days of infusion treatment, which means three days of being hooked up to an IV for eight hours straight, getting massive amounts of pain medication injected straight into my veins—the goal being to help bust through the awful pain cycle of constant headache and give my brain a chance to rest.

The infusion center is located on the same floor as the headache center, and each patient receiving infusion treatment, whether for chemo or for migraine headaches, is placed in a room with a comfortable reclining chair. My neurologist has told me to arrive by 8 A.M. and expect to be there until 3 or 4 in the afternoon. I'm allowed to have my phone with me during the treatment process, so I queue up podcasts to ready myself for the long day. The first day of treatment, I'm assigned a nurse who seems quite strict. She has a Germanic accent and doesn't smile or make small talk, but as a non-smiler myself who fails regularly at small talk, I try not to take that as a bad sign. She checks my vitals and seems mildly curious about my diagnosis of CSF leak, which she has never heard of before, but quickly moves on to explaining the process to me. Basically, I will sit in a reclining chair and be hooked up to an IV. I will be given a series of medications, in a specific order, normally designed for migraine patients. Some of these medications will be for pain, some for inflammation (in other words, more steroids). They will be administered in a cycle, so each dose will be repeated twice throughout the day. I will likely sleep through most of it, thanks to the diphenhydramine and lorazepam they will give me (basically, Benadryl and Ativan), and then, once the medications have all been administered via IV, I will be free to go home. This process will be repeated for two more days, for a total of three days in a row of headache attack meds. Then I will need to continue taking a course of steroids, tapering off over the course of a week. And then, theoretically, my head pain will improve—if not the leak headache itself, which of course these medications are not able to fix, then the secondary, overall headache I have from having the leak for so long.

Once I change into the requisite gown and no-slip socks, I return to the recliner and am handed paperwork about the medicine I will be given. I am to sign each packet, one for each medication, to indicate I understand the risks. Diphenhydramine and lorazepam I am familiar with; many of the others I have not yet encountered.

Prochlorperazine. Treats severe nausea and vomiting. Also treats schizophrenia. This medicine may cause the following problems: Tardive dyskinesia (a muscle disorder that could become permanent), neuroleptic malignant syndrome (a nerve disorder that could be life-threatening).

Valproate sodium. Treats seizures. Possible side effects: blistering, peeling, red skin rash; sudden and severe stomach pain.

Methylprednisone. A steroid. Treats inflammation. This medicine may cause mood or behavior changes.

Magnesium sulfate. Prevents seizures, especially in pregnant women with severe toxemia.

Dihydroergotamine. Also known as DHE. Treats migraine headaches. Possible side effects: chest pain, confusion, sudden or severe headache. This medicine may cause the following problems: risk of heart attack or heart rhythm problems; increased blood pressure; higher risk of stroke.

If I have any negative reactions to any of these, the nurse tells me, we can remove it from the infusion cycle. "Do people often have negative reactions?" I ask. Her face remains neutral as she tells me, "DHE can be difficult. But we can talk about that when it's time. Now, what would you like for lunch? We are allowed to order you a sandwich from Subway."

I sign the papers, indicating my understanding, request a turkey sandwich with yellow mustard, and recline the chair as far back as it can go. The nurse brings me warm blankets and dims the lights, and once the IV is placed, I begin to drift off in a haze of lorazepam and diphenhydramine, listening to a podcast on the history of the English language.

From time to time, the nurse reappears, swapping out an IV bag for the next medicine and making sure I'm doing okay. Every once in a while, she rechecks my blood pressure. I am groggy for most of this, and don't really notice any reactions to the medications I'm being given. Before the DHE, however, the nurse comes and sits by my side. "Now," she says, looking even more stern than usual, "this medicine you're about to have administered. Some people have very strong reactions. For some people, they say it feels as though they are having a heart attack. It narrows blood vessels, which for some people helps them, but for others can feel uncomfortable."

"I don't think I want to do this," I say, but I'm sleepy, and not putting up much of a fight.

"How about this," she says. "I will stay with you while the medicine is administered, and if you feel uncomfortable from the effects of it, we can remove it from the afternoon cycle of medicine and not include it over the next two days."

I nod, and she puts the bag of DHE onto the IV stand and does what she needs to do with my IV to start the medicine flowing. She sits down next to me and holds my hands, looking directly into my eyes. "It will take a few minutes," she says, "but if you feel bad, just squeeze my hands. Okay?"

"Okay," I say, and together we wait.

It doesn't take too long for me to begin to feel something. "My chest feels a little tight," I tell her, but what's really terrifying is what happens next: My entire brain begins to feel tight. But not just tight; it's like my brain is suffocating. It feels as though it's being squeezed from the inside out, like someone is siphoning all the liquid from inside it, like there's a liquid center that's rapidly being sucked out. "Oh god, my head," I say, and start to cry. The scraping headache I've felt for so long—the one I always describe to my neurologists as feeling like someone's taking a melon baller and scraping out the inside of my skull; this is exactly what that feels like, except all over my brain, instead of just the bottom of it. My heart is racing, and my chest feels tight and my brain feels tight, and I'm squeezing the nurse's hands as tightly as my brain is squeezing from the medicine, and she's telling me I'm going to be okay, that it's almost done, that we don't have to do it again, it's just the narrowing of blood vessels, the pain of constriction, and it will be over soon.

And then it is. I'm given more lorazepam, more diphenhydramine. Tissues to wipe my tears. The nurse tells me we'll skip the second dose of DHE scheduled for the afternoon, and that she'll make a note to not include it in the list of meds for tomorrow and the next day. She brings me my Subway sandwich, and I eat it awkwardly, trying not to bend my IV elbow too much, and then I retreat into the haze of the relaxation drugs as I await my second round.

When it's over, I take a cab home and sleep until it's time to wake up the next morning and do it all over again. Show up, change clothes, sign forms, get IV, settle into recliner with blankets, drift off in a drug haze, eat a Subway sandwich, fall asleep to more podcasts, groggily find my way home, and do it all over again for one more day.

After that, I take steroids for another five days to taper off the bolus I've been given during the days of infusion. I don't like how these steroids make me feel. The dexamethasone I took before made me productive, even if that productivity was ill-advised; but the prednisone makes me angry. I hate everything. Luckily, I am also sleepy for most of the time I'm on the tapering course, sleeping off the three days of groggy medications, sleeping my way back into the fog. So my anger is limited in scope somewhat. It's hard to be irritated in dreams.

Weeks later, my overall headache pain has been improved by the infusion treatment, but the leak headache is still there, meaning that if I'm upright, my head hurts, and of course the brain fog is a constant companion. My routine now is to mostly lie in bed, doing light chores and minimal activity in the mornings when I'm clearer, and trying to be more horizontal at the end of the day, when everything seems harder. When I lie there, in bed, I wonder if this is just how it's going to be for the rest of my life. The last time I spoke with the neurologist, she told me that even if the hospital had the diagnostic tools to find the source of the leak, they wouldn't be able to fix it. "No one here can do it," she tells me, leading me to wonder: *Why the hell am I here then?*

23

December 2015

I'm in my neurologist's office, crying, because this is what I do now, even though I know this will be codified in my file as Depression, Recurrent, Mild. And yet I can't go on like this. I can't keep coming to appointments and filling out forms and answering the same questions—*Are there any events that have affected your headache? Have your headache symptoms or location changed?*—when the problem is that I am leaking cerebrospinal fluid and no one can help me.

"I need to be fixed," I tell her. "I can't live like this, just treating the symptoms."

She hands me a tissue and makes a note in my file and tells me that actually, she just attended a neurology conference and heard a really fascinating talk given by this doctor from Duke University, in North Carolina. This doctor, who's a neuroradiologist, gave a presentation about treating a patient with a spinal CSF leak, and my neurologist was thinking the whole time, *This sounds just like my patient!* She tells me that I should call this doctor at Duke and set up a time for a visit; that, from what it sounded like, this doctor's team of neuroradiologists could help me.

"Do you need to give me a referral, or get in touch with them, or, how does the process work?" I ask, but she says no, she will give me a referral to send, but I have to call them myself. This doesn't make sense to me, and also makes me less likely to do it. "Won't they take it more seriously if the call comes from a doctor?" But she says that's not how it works, and that it's fine, and that if I just google the doctor's name, her information will show up and I can call the number listed for her at Duke. That seems like a lot of work for a person whose brain isn't working well, but I take down the woman's name: Dr. Linda Gray-Leithe.

Her name has turned up in my internet searches before, along with the other doctor of last resort, in California, Dr. Schievink, and when I search specifically for her and Duke University and spinal CSF leaks and how to contact her, I find glowing mentions of her and her team on obscure forums and bulletin boards. *Dr. Gray saved my life*, people write. *Dr. Gray is amazing. The entire staff at Duke is incredible. Changed my life. Sealed and healed.*

I find the website with her contact information, and eventually I get up the nerve to call. It seems insane, to call from Philadelphia and say I need an appointment with a doctor in Durham. My voice when I finally make the call is entirely uptalk and apology, even my hello and introduction are performed as an upward glissando of question marks. And yet the intake person seems not only *not* confounded or confused, but almost bored by what I have to say. He cuts me off, thankfully, before I can waver too long in my awkward apologetic request to be seen, and tells me they're already making appointments for mid-January by this point and he would be happy to schedule me. He doesn't question me, doesn't wonder at why I, a patient, might be calling, and from so far away. He just tells me his name is Horace, and that I need to send him all my records: all my MRIs, all my CT scans, all my medical letters and doctor's notes and printouts from hospital visits; everything I can possibly send that documents my experience with the leak. He does mention that Dr. Gray's schedule is full for the foreseeable future, but assures me that one of her associates will be able to see me in January, probably a doctor by the name of Peter Kranz. I take down the address where these things should be mailed, and note Horace's direct line in case of further questions, and then I begin the process of assembling the required records.

It is a challenge. Some things I have saved from my visits and can make copies of; other things I can access online and print out. Still other things I must request from various medical records departments, and pick up in person so as to expedite the process, which could otherwise take weeks. I take cab rides, lying down in backseats, and procure DVDs of my scans from two different hospitals. I assemble a packet of all the things I have gathered, and write a cover letter including all of my contact information and insurance information and as brief a summary as possible of my medical history as it pertains to the leak, and mail it to Duke.

In a week or so, it's all returned to me, in an envelope with a Duke return address, no cover letter, no note, just all the information I'd sent them sent back to me. I wonder whether or not this means they have rejected me as a potential patient. Maybe my scans are as unremarkable to Dr. Gray's team as they are to everyone else who's seen them. I consider calling Horace to find out if there's anything else I need to do, but then just before Christmas, I get a phone call from one of Dr. Gray's associates, Dr. Kranz.

It's evening, I've been lying on the floor of the family room with the kids while they watch TV, and so I go upstairs to take the phone call in the half darkness of the living room, lying down again on the couch, so nervous my teeth are chattering as he asks me to give a synopsis of my history, so relieved to hear him tell me that, after looking through my information and reviewing the scans and hearing about my symptoms, he thinks he can help. Not just help my symptoms, but possibly, hopefully, seal this leak. This seems almost impossible to believe, and I try hard to keep my voice steady as I ask, "Are you sure?" But he is sure.

He tells me a scheduler will call in a few days to set up a time for me to come there. It'll be a two-day outpatient procedure—some diagnostic tests performed on the first day, then patching treatment on the second—so I should plan to stay in a hotel near the hospital. It will take several days afterward before it will be safe for me to travel home. I should budget for a four- or five-day stay total, conservatively, if everything goes well.

He tells me about a private Facebook group that exists for people dealing with CSF leaks, many of whom are in the process of being treated at Duke, or who have already been treated at Duke. He recommends joining and reaching out, looking there for recommendations about hotels and travel tips, and reading through people's experiences of their procedures at his clinic. He tells me the group was founded by patients, and that while he himself isn't personally a member, he knows that it functions as much as a source of information as a source of support and camaraderie. I'm not much of a joiner, or a group person, really, but something about his earnestness makes me jot down the info in the scribble of notes I've been taking during the call, makes me promise to look into it, makes me promise to join. I am teary with thanks by the end of the call, and nervously exhilarated. For the first time in a long time I'm feeling a thing I thought I'd forgotten how to feel.

Hope.

24

I used to be an early adopter. My dad, a computer guy by vocation and avocation, let my grade-school-aged sisters and me fool around on his just-for-fun Radio Shack TRS-80 long before most people had machines in their homes. I remember popping in cassette tapes of computer programs, the day he showed me the wonders of 10 PRINT "HELLO WORLD!" 20 GOTO 10. I was on the internet back when it was called the Web, capitalized, and always proceeded by the words *World Wide*; on forums back when they were still called bulletin boards; in instant messaging groups back when they were still called chat rooms and no user ever used their actual name as their user name. I posted, I lurked, I surfed; I eventually forsook Lycos and Infoseek and AltaVista for something called Google. I blogged.

But after Nate's accident as a toddler, I mostly stopped writing on the internet about my life. It was an abrupt thing, at first, in the wake of what had happened; and then a gradual thing, a choice I made to curtail the amount of information I shared and the frequency with which I shared it. I was conflicted about writing about motherhood online as my children grew older, anyway, and the stories about my life with them no longer seemed solely mine to tell. Eventually I stepped back, as the demands of my non-virtual life eclipsed my internet-based one, and, for the first time, let technology pass me by.

I watched as social media transformed the internet into an entirely new space, one where real names were the norm and anonymity was the odd exception. Where the ubiquitousness of internet-connected phones and specialized applications made networks of consciousness emerge, real-time communities forming around world events or even local events. I watched from a distance as my listserv friends became Yahoo Group friends and then Gmail friends and then MySpace friends, and then Facebook friends with each other; began vlogging instead of blogging; joined a thing called Twitter, a thing called Tumblr, a thing called Instagram, a thing called Pinterest. I watched from close-up as my kids began to participate in their own subset of the internet. I joined Twitter in 2010, as a capitulation to the reality of publishers encouraging authors to have some sort of social media presence. But other than that, I stayed on the sidelines.

And so, when the doctor from North Carolina suggested I join the private CSF Leak Facebook group, I'd hesitated. I'd resisted the urge to assimilate for ten years—could I really relent now, after all this time? And yet it sounded as though this community he'd mentioned could prove to be extremely useful. The little internet searching I'd done had yielded forum posts here and there, many of them years old; nothing like an active community of users, sharing current information and support. How amazing would it be to find other people going through what I was going through—how amazing would it be to feel less alone? The thought of that reminds me of the early days of writing about motherhood on the internet, connecting with other women all over the world, all of us writing in isolation about what turned out, we discovered, to be a profoundly shared event. And so I tentatively decide to enter the vortex, submitting to the social media behemoth that seems to now define the modern online experience, and finally joining the rest of the world on Facebook. But I do it the way it used to be done in the "olden days" of the internet: under a pseudonym.

The CSF leak group is instantly welcoming, and at first I mostly lurk, reading through the files and documents that members have compiled over the years containing everything from people's personal stories about living with CSF leaks to tips about travel, hotel information, which numbers to call, which doctors are responsive, links to medical journal articles and informative websites, suggestions of things to bring with you when you go for tests and procedures, people's experiences with those procedures. The sheer amount of practical advice about how to manage daily life when you can't be upright for long makes the group worthwhile: I learn about the benefits of Spanx and other compression clothes, which kinds of caffeinated drinks have the most caffeine, what foods can affect intracranial pressure, how you can save yourself from the grossness of lying on a doctor's office floor, or a floor anywhere you have to go, by bringing a yoga mat with you, a small travel pillow, a light blanket.

The board is full of stories. Everyone has a narrative they've honed, after telling it to doctors for years, in some cases; but there is a relief in telling this particular kind of story to a group of listeners who know exactly what you're talking about. The people here know all the plot twists—the failed blood patches, the skeptical doctors, the havoc wreaked on marriages, on families, on careers; the arcane variations—underlying conditions like Marfan syndrome, like Ehlers-Danlos syndrome, like postural orthostatic tachycardia syndrome, like Chiari malformation, like idiopathic intracranial hypertension, like having shunts placed and having your dura shaved down, and pieces of skull removed; the dark nights of the soul—hopelessness and depression and pain, addiction, distress, job loss; and the possibility of happy endings—those who are "sealed and healed" and return to the boards with tales of strange worlds: sitting upright without a headache, being able to think and work and exercise and live the way we all used to in the Before Times.

The worst-case scenario stories scare me; the happy-ending stories give me fragile hope. I lurk and read and come to recognize the daily posters, the regulars, those who always encourage no matter how desperate their own situation, those who are desperate beyond all encouragement, those who are struggling, and those who are able to help in the midst of their own struggles. Despite my natural shyness about joining groups in general, I come to see that my story is a story like many others there, that I belong there, and so I post and I am welcomed. I comment and receive "likes." I adopt the vocabulary of the boards. I am a leaker. I make friends with another leaker whose sense of humor always comes through in her posts, who's scheduled to be treated at Duke just weeks after I'm going to be there. We begin to message each other off-site, through Messenger and then via text. She used to be a lawyer; I used to be a writer. We are brain-compromised; there are typos, run-on sentences, confusion. And yet we understand each other.

There are characters in this group, like in any online group. One guy who joins the group around the same time as me is somewhat my opposite: He joins under his real name, he's gregarious and outgoing, and posts videos of himself almost daily. His videos are sometimes funny and sometimes sad, as he shares his frustration about this new constant headache he's battling and the lack of help he's getting from the doctors he's seeing. He isn't sure he has a leak, but everyone on the board is sympathetic to his situation, as everyone on there, old-timers and newcomers alike, knows what it's like to be in pain and not be taken seriously. Miraculously, he manages to get an appointment at Duke only weeks into his strange headaches, and weeks sooner than many of us who called far earlier and are still awaiting our appointments. There are some people on the board who have suffered with their leaks for over a decade. Others have been treated multiple times, undergoing surgery after surgery, and are still not healed. Others are in the process of recovery, but even those optimistic posts are tentative and full of doubt. So we all watch with curiosity and excitement tinged with a little bit of envy as we follow his progress: his journey to Duke, his test results, the disappointing news that no leak was seen on his imaging, the perplexing news that the doctors there do not think he has a leak at all, that his headaches are caused by something else. "I've loved being a part of this group," he says in one of his last videos. "I may still hang out here while I figure out what's going on with me." Everyone encourages him to stay, to keep sharing. The videos of him sitting upright, walking around, being vertical, being goofy, cheer everyone up. But he doesn't end up sticking around for too long.

Later, this guy will ask to video chat with me after I return from Duke, to talk to me about my experience there, and I will, even though I am high on opiates and weighted down by the steel pipe that is my spine, filled with blood clotting along my dura. "I hope this is it for you," he will tell me, "I really hope you're healed. And if you are—man, just run away from this group, from all these groups, and don't look back." I think he means to convey some kind of message of empowerment, like, *If you're better, stay better, and don't dwell on the past once you're headache-free*; but still, it sounds ominous. I understand his longing to not have to identify as a sick person, as a person belonging to a group of sick people. And I understand how these things work: The people who heal, who recover, eventually leave; the people who are struggling stay. Sometimes people who recover end up relapsing and return to the group. Sometimes people who are recovered find it hard to leave the community that's been such a part of their lives for so long, and become mentors and cheerleaders of a sort, posting hopeful messages, providing support. But after going through this by myself for so long, this community feels like a balm to me, not a conflict, not a burden. Not someplace to flee.

Just after I get the call from Dr. Kranz, about a week or so after I join the group, I get a letter in the mail, a thick envelope from the City of Philadelphia. I know what it is before I open it, but it's still a shock. My divorce is final: These are the papers making it official. I text Gil to let him know that it's here—he was sent his own copy, at my address, formerly *our* address—and he comes over to get it.

"This is it?" he says, and I say, "This is it." We both hold our separate copies of the divorce decree, standing in the foyer as the kids sit in the other room, doing homework, listening to music. Neither of us is sure what to do—what's the protocol, after all, for the official ending of a twenty-year marriage, the transition from life partners to co-parents?

"Well, congrats, I guess," I say, and we both kind of laugh, and then we hug each other, tearfully. This is the right decision, we have both agreed. But still it has been a hard decision. It feels bittersweet to suddenly, officially, be on the other side of this process.

"Congrats," he says, before leaving.

Within weeks, I will be removed from our health insurance, just in time for my trip to Duke.

25

There is more space when it's just us, the three of us, me and Emi and Nate. Gone are the piles of mail and unread medical journals, the boxes of papers, the hoard of things to be organized, the task of organizing them put off and put off until finally the hoard is just a hoard, a series of towering piles inside a room that used to be a bedroom but now is a holding place for this stuff that hasn't been looked at for years. Now that room is a bedroom again, now the piles and files and papers and boxes and clothes and the unfiltered history of a life has been transported to a new house, a new place for it all to take root, to vine, the pruning of which is no longer my problem.

The day he moved out, I'd wrapped myself in layers of compression—bike shorts over bike shorts over Spanx—to force my cerebrospinal fluid upward, giving me buoyancy, and I'd walked to a store to buy curtains for the living room. It seemed, to my half-functioning brain, the right thing to do. I needed to absent myself from the scene at the house, the movers and his parents there physically dismantling the proof of our cohabitation, the literal removal of him from our shared space. I needed air, I needed space as the emptiness of the house slowly revealed itself, as his parents quailed with emotion I wasn't up to the task of managing, as he and I gamely agreed upon last-minute questions of ownership over small items we hadn't considered until now, when we were faced with the prospect of losing them.

We'd lived in the house for seven years by that point, and we still didn't have curtains in the living room. It's true that the light was nice, that it was pleasing to have the sun streaming through on bright days, that even when it was overcast the room was filled with light, that that side of the house faces a narrow street not much larger than an alleyway, with no neighbor windows looking into ours. But the real reason we'd never gotten curtains was that he'd wanted to be a part of the process of choosing them, and he'd never had time. I'd bought some once, just simple, inexpensive things, just to have them, just to try, but he'd vetoed them; he wanted to choose them together, and we would do that someday, when he had time. But he never had time. For seven years.

I walked to the store, walked away from the process taking place of our house becoming my house, and felt my head throbbing with every step. I said *curtains* to myself, over and over, so I wouldn't forget my mission, and then I was there, in the store, surrounded by all kinds of pleasing furniture, all arranged with no piles of mail on the tables, or clothes on the floor, or papers covering every available surface. There was no realistic tableaux of how a busy person might actually use these furnishings, and I realized that was because this was aspirational, a showroom floor, a kind of lie about real life; and yet I also wanted to aspire. I found the curtains I wanted, found four packs of them for the living room windows. There was some closet at home, I was sure of it, that held fixtures for hanging, purchased long ago during one of my attempts to make curtains happen, before I'd given up. Around me, in the calculated beauty of simulated living rooms, anxious couples bickered about rugs and end tables, men sat defeated on couches, women rolled their eyes as they stalked off toward the dinnerware. By now, at home, the furniture he was taking with him to his new place must be loaded up into the truck. At some point I would have to come back here and pick out a table, all by myself, no partner to argue with about the virtues of chairs versus a long bench, midcentury modern versus rustic. But the curtains were the first step, for now. I took them to the counter, and the woman asked "Will that be all?" and I said, "That will be everything."

Now the curtains hang in the living room, now there is a table with benches instead of chairs in the dining room, now the house is emptied of papers and boxes and tension. In some ways, the space of just the three of us reminds me of when the kids were very little and he was in medical school. Some weeks, it would just be the three of us for days at a time, and during the rare moments he was home, he was either asleep or studying, so he might as well have been gone, as the daily routine of toddler and preschooler life continued, immune to his presence or absence. In those days, like now, I was alone with them most of the time, and there were no vacation days, no sick days, no days off. I was on a permanent, 24/7 call schedule, and if I had limitations due to my own work that needed to be done (somehow, in the brief moments when they were asleep) or due to illness, I had to get creative.

One particular winter, when I was incapacitated by the flu and a nagging back injury, exacerbated by picking up a squirming toddler, I came up with a number of what Emi and Nate called "lying down games" to help fill the long hours of solo parenting. One of these games, which we called "Covers," was played as follows: 1. Lie on the bed, then pull the covers up over everyone's heads while everyone yells "Covers!" 2. Stay under the covers as long as possible until one of you panics and yells "No covers!" 3. Repeat until weary. Another big hit was "No-Water-Bath," which involved playing with toys in the bathtub without any water—the bonus for the incapacitated adult being that there is no slippery child to have to pick up afterward, plus the relief of being able to lie on the cool floor of the bathroom, occasionally interjecting statements like "Uh-huh, that's great!" or "Wow!" to fulfill your role as Game Master. "Tiny Swimming Pools" was also a favorite, requiring only a non-wood-based floor and every shape and size of plastic container, filled halfway full with water, for them to have their tiny toys swim in (bonus: clean floor afterward). And then there was Nate's invention, "Surprise Toys," which required me to lie down on some comfortable surface and say, "I *really* hope nobody comes over here and puts their toys on me while I'm taking this nap! That would be *quite* a surprise!" and then pretend to fall asleep while he and/or Emi placed small toys all over my body. Then, after a blessed five minutes or so of rest, with them barely able to contain their laughter in anticipation of what would come next, I would have to "wake up," realize that there were small toys balanced all over me, and say, "What?! Oh no! TOYS!" The game would end when, in that moment of pretend toy-panic, the toys would become dislodged from their positions and fall off me. And then, of course, it would start again.

They are no longer that little, and no longer as easily distracted by my attempts to ameliorate the fact that this lying down game is my life now. I want to shield them from the reality of my exhaustion and pain the same way I did when they were younger, making the best of it, normalizing it, turning it into something fun. When they were younger, when they were toddlers, the thought of adults having needs was nearly developmentally impossible, and my attempts at consistency and calm despite whatever was going on with me personally helped ground them, helped give them a solid base from which to learn to cope with their own needs. Now, too, as teens, the idea of adults being weak or having needs is scary and overwhelming—this is why the scorn, the disdain, when the cracks begin to show, when you realize the so-called grown-ups around you are as clueless as everyone else, that this competence is all a charade. The charade is still important; it's still important for me to try to be consistent and calm, to model things for them, which is also a way of modeling things for myself. However, it's also important for me to allow them to see a little of the effort it takes to do that.

And so I embrace the space that's left when he is gone, I let us fill it together. I am playing the lying down game all the time, but I try to play it near them, lying down with them while they do homework, lying down with them while they watch TV or play video games, lying down with them while they hang out with me in my bed, telling me stories about school and friends and funny things that happened on the internet. I worry that they might feel lost in all this space, that they might feel a sense of abandonment with their dad moving out, with me unable to be as physically present and active as I always have been with them. And yet they also need this space right now; even without this massive change in our family structure, even without this illness to cut me off from real life, they would be changing, becoming more independent, more self-sufficient. This is age-appropriate, normal; and yet I worry at how it intersects with this jarring shift in their lives.

There is a comfort in this new routine, though, in how it returns us to the way things were before, just the three of us, before the time when there was tension and grief and worry and sadness and guilt and anger about it being just the three of us. Now it is the relief of just the three of us, coming up with ways to fill the days together, being creative about the fact that I need to be lying down most of the time.

How to remain lying down while in the process of getting to Duke for my procedure is a game I haven't figured out the rules of just yet. Flying seems impossible: I understand the physics involved in flight, but the physics involved in my getting myself into a cab and then standing up and walking through the airport and then sitting through the flight, unable to lie down, and then standing again and then getting another cab and then getting to the hotel seem impossible to understand or execute at a time when my cumulative daily functional upright time is measured in minutes.

More than that, when I ask about whether or not I can do this all alone—theoretically survive a flight, take cabs to and from the hospital for my tests and procedures, recover at the hotel, and get myself back to Philadelphia after five days or so, if all goes well— the doctor says absolutely not. I need to have a person with me; this is not something I can do alone. I check in with the leakers in the Facebook group, and they all concur. And yet who can I impose upon to do this with me? I can't ask Gil, as he will need to be with the kids during the time I'm gone, and also because spending five days in a hotel room with me while I'm incapacitated is likely the last thing he wants to do at this point; his parents have kindly offered to help in whatever way I need, but I can't possibly ask them to do this, mainly due to the awkwardness of sharing a hotel room and being cared for for five days by people who are now my ex-in-laws, and also because it is too much of an imposition, too much to ask.

It feels too much to ask of my sister Jessie, too, but when I tell her I am to be treated at Duke, she arranges for the time off and says she will drive me to North Carolina, take me to my appointments, stay with me while I recover, and drive me back home again. I can lie down for the seven-hour car ride, and I do. We make our way through seven hours of true-crime podcasts and conversation, a cooler loaded with snacks and drinks within arm's reach as I lie fully reclined in the passenger seat, and I'm grateful to not have to do this alone, grateful to not have to hold this fragile hope all by myself as we get closer and closer to the place that may offer me some relief, finally, that may even possibly, unbelievably, unimaginably provide a true end to the lying down game.

26

This is what I do when I am startled, or confronted by an argument: I freeze. If I can become very still and wait it out, become invisible, then it will stop, and I will be safe.

This is not a great strategy for dealing with confrontation. And yet it is a powerful reflex, one against which I have to actively work to fight in a moment when I find myself in a combative conversation or stressful dynamic. This is why I end up staying longer than I intend to, or agreeing to things I don't necessarily want to do, or losing an argument I should win. This is not a pattern that works in my favor in the long run.

My marriage has been a long argument, and I am perpetually freezing. It's true that over the years I have gotten better at responding, at not holding myself so still that I can barely breathe.

And it's true that when the argument is about something that's not me, when it's about the kids and what's right for them, for instance, I am able to resist the urge to hide and instead fight on their behalf, or for what I know is the right thing. But my first instinct is always to not break, to not allow myself to shatter. And so often, against my better judgment, I agree, I soothe, I capitulate. I freeze.

I think about this, as I lie in bed, frozen in place by my leaky brain fluid. Have I been choosing this? Is this another way to hide? Am I resisting the stress of my life, of my shattered marriage, by lying here, hiding in place, a kind of pain-riddled, cognitively impaired Snow White in a glass coffin, waiting for someone to wake me up?

The kids think I am under glass, for the most part. Shut away in my room, in the dark, lying still, not moving. They see me sometimes, surprising them by being upright for a moment, massaging the back of my head, wincing; but that's just another thing grown-ups do to be annoying, like complaining about dumb grown-up things that don't matter. *Headaches. Taxes. Traffic. Those darn kids.* I'm a sitcom mom clutching my head, complaining, frowning over a laugh track. This pain is a thing I am doing to them, or doing to avoid them, or to inconvenience them. I haven't told them how serious or scary it is, because I don't know whether it's truly scary or serious, and because I don't want to make them worry. So I allow them to find it vaguely irritating. *Of course* I can't go to the store, or run an errand, *of course* I can't take them to a friend's house—ugh, *moms*. But I see their anxiety, slightly, just beneath their evolutionarily protective buffer of normal, developmentally appropriate teenaged narcissism. I see them wondering, nervously: *What is really going on?*

I have protected them from my pain, because pain is so impersonal, so pointless, when it's happening to someone else. Hearing about someone else's pain is like hearing about someone else's dream: It's diffuse and nonspecific, no matter how detail-rich the dreamer's description; always more immediate for the dreamer, more theoretical to the person hearing about the dream. And so they understand that I'm in pain, but that pain is abstract for them in the way someone else's pain is always abstract, and in the way that parental pain seems particularly impossible. My pain floats around them like a bad dream, intractable, undefinable, and ultimately irrelevant.

They know—of course I have told them—that I somehow have a tear somewhere in the thing covering my spine, the same thing they have covering their spines, that keeps cerebrospinal fluid in its proper place. They know that this is causing a slow leak, that my brain, unlike theirs, doesn't have the cushion of fluid it should in order to function properly. They don't know fully why, because I don't fully know why. I am through the looking-glass, unable to communicate how strange and nonsensical things are from here.

Nate has a daily journal he's required to keep for a class in school. He shows me one of his entries from when I first got sick. It reads:

5/6/15. My mom is going through a tough time right now. Here's what's going on. A month or so back my mom was getting constant headaches. It went on for a few weeks, until my mom saw a doctor and found out that brain juice is spilling out of her brain. Imagine a half-full bottle. When it stands up, the liquid is at the bottom, but when it's on its side, it evens out. That pretty much explains what my mom has to do, just lie down.

Here he has drawn a diagram, a glass bottle standing upright, half full, all the liquid pooled at the bottom; and next to it, a glass bottle on its side, the liquid distributed along the length of it. This is exactly how I've explained it to him, my need to be flat, so that cerebrospinal fluid can reach my brain. His entry continues:

And, on top of alllllllllll that, my parents are getting divorced.

There's a lot of pain I'm trying to keep from them. But it doesn't work like that. It seeps out, amorphous and uncontainable. I just want their pain to be their own pain, a pain I can help them process. I don't want them to have to take on the burden of mine. And so I hold myself very still, and try to let them see only the smooth surface, reflecting back at them what they need.

One night, incapacitated by pain, dizzy with the inability to think, I am confounded by the simple process of getting out of bed and making dinner for the kids. This is before Gil has moved out, but he has long been absent, and so I think: *Where is their father?* I don't know. But I can't get up, and the kids are hungry, and even lying flat I hurt so much I can't think, and I see text messages from them that say things like, "Food??? Hello??????"

I reply to Emi. I type, assisted by autocorrect: "My head is really bad right now. I'll order a pizza. When the doorbell rings, just answer it and give the pizza guy the $20 that's on the table." I'm about to try to find the pizza number when she writes back: "No."

"???" I respond.

"I'm not comfortable interacting with strangers," she writes.

"I'm not comfortable with brain fluid leaking out of my brain," I reply.

This isn't fair of me. She doesn't know how bad this is. I have protected her, I've protected both of them, from how bad this is.

I see the three dots hovering, disappearing, hovering, disappearing. They don't come back. There's no response.

Where is their father?

I order the pizza. I get out of bed. By the time I make my way to the first floor, my head is pounding, throbbing. The static circle of pain at the base of my skull on the right side of my head is a ring of fire, searing me; the rest of my head throbs with my heartbeat. I sit on the stairs, weeping, because that's what happens when I'm upright now, tears streaming from my eyes even though I'm not sad, exactly, and I wait for the pizza to arrive, thinking to myself, *This isn't their fault, they don't know, I haven't told them this is bad, or serious, I've tried to protect them from this, I've let them think I'm annoying rather than really sick because that's easier, but maybe it's not, maybe this is like the divorce, maybe this is a thing they shouldn't be blindsided by, except I don't have any words of reassurance about this, because I have no idea when this will end or what the prognosis is or how to break the glass in case of emergency.*

The pizza guy shows up and I remember to give him the money, the way I'd instructed Emi, and I don't even care that I must seem to him to be obviously distraught and crying and pained and con-fused, I just take the food and close the door and bring the pizza to where Emi is and let her see me, distraught and crying and pained and confused, and I start to say, "I'm sorry, this is serious, and I know it's scary—" but she cuts me off and asks, "Where's Daddy?"

I don't know.

The pain is so bad I feel like I might vomit, and so I go back upstairs, leaving her to deal with plates and napkins and glasses and drinks and sharing the food with Nate, and get back into bed, as flat as possible, waiting out the worst of the pain, waiting for a bit of relief that may or may not come after being flat for an hour, to counteract the fifteen minutes I was up, lying very, very still, as still as glass, and hoping this is not a thing that will break me.

There was a time when glass was a new technology. We don't tend to think of glass as something technological now, as we exist in a world where glass is pervasive, commonplace, and unremarkable. But there was a time when it was new, and its mysterious nature was a source of fascination for people. It's transparent, yet solid. It connects us—there, visible, is the world outside the window—and yet separates us—there is the window. It can be a vessel: Hold it carefully and you can drink from it. And yet it is fragile: Become careless and it shatters. It can magnify, and it can shrink. It can focus light and also diffuse it. It can reflect, allowing you to see yourself, and can also let light pass through, making things visible, allowing you to see past yourself.

As the technology of glass began to become more widespread and accessible to people, it brought with it the paranoia that always seems to accompany new technology, no matter when its invention. In the late Middle Ages in Europe, this took the form of what came to be called the "glass delusion," a very specific kind of depression and anxiety in which the sufferer believed themselves to be made of glass. A person afflicted with the glass delusion became fearful of movement, as they worried they might shatter, and coped with this by wearing layers and layers of clothes, or carrying pillows with them wherever they went, or remaining very, very still. The French king Charles VI was said to suffer from this, and refused to let people touch him, lest he shatter into a million pieces.

I feel an empathy for these glass people, the way they feared they couldn't move or else they would break open, the way their chosen metaphor was so transparent. This is what I do, too: I reflect back at people what they want to see. I focus the light on others, becoming the conduit for someone else's clarity. Or I take in the light and refract it, separating a beam of light into a spectrum of colors, illuminating a previously unseen reality. I, too, become a complicated thing that's easy to take for granted, that's strong but vulnerable, that people forget about the fragility of until it finally shatters.

"Why do you need a lawyer?" my husband asks, early into our separation process. "This is something we can figure out together, there's no need to make it complicated, we can have an amicable divorce." But I remind him that this is how this has always worked, that when he has an argument in mind, he voices it, and I freeze, and he wears me down until I give in or say yes just to make the arguing stop. I remind him that this is what happens with us, even when things are amicable. "You always win," I tell him. "I need someone to argue for me. I need to have someone to help me fight instead of giving up." This is me trying to unfreeze, and he concedes, finally, letting me win this small battle.

My marriage is a kind of Cinderella's glass slipper I have tiptoed around in, ever mindful that stepping too hard or too carelessly could break it, lodge a splinter of glass in my foot. I'm hobbled either way.

He shows up one night after work, months into my illness, home for a rare moment, and comes into my dark room, flipping on the lights, startling me. "What do you want me to do?" he asks. I'm confused by the question. I don't even know how to begin to answer it. He hasn't been here for days, I can't be upright, even lying flat the pain never goes away, I can't do anything. It's not even a question of what I want him to do; I need him to do everything. Anything. Parent his children. Feed the cats. Clean the litter boxes. Take care of the house. Make food. Get the mail. Dust, vacuum, take out garbage, wipe counters. "I don't know," I say, unable to articulate any of this, the indignity of being unable to do things, the indignity of having to explain the basic concepts of living in a household, the indignity of being myself helpless and still having to help. "Look around," I say. "Pick something. Do it." He nods, says "Okay," then just stands there. After a while he says, "I hope you start to get better." I begin to say, "Me too," feeling the relief of some brief compassion, until he continues: "Because we really need to get this divorce settled."

The way we think about ourselves protects us.

The way we think about ourselves becomes a reality that we protect.

There is an account from 1561 of a Parisian patient suffering from the glass delusion who was, himself, a glassmaker. Aware of the power and fragility of his creation, he became entranced by it, and was convinced that he, himself, was the literal embodiment of the glass he made. Fearful of shattering, he carried a pillow with him wherever he went, to sit on, in case the movement of lowering himself to sit would cause him to splinter into a thousand shards.

Imagine, the glassmaker himself, imprisoned by his conception of himself as a glass man, a kind of human glass prism.

But he found himself cured when his physician visited one day and gave him what was described as a "severe thrashing." When the glassmaker cried out in pain, the doctor asked him if it hurt. And when the glassmaker replied it did, the light finally shone through him as he realized that if it hurt, then he could not truly be made of glass. Because, whatever else its qualities, glass cannot feel pain.

The glass delusion was a way to protect himself from pain. From feeling vulnerable.

If he's glass, he feels no pain.

If he's glass, he doesn't have to suffer.

This is the story I tell Emi when she comes to me, terrified, in December, nine months into my illness, three months after her dad moving out, the month the divorce was final, weeks before I was to go to North Carolina to, hopefully, be cured. She's freezing, she says—not cold, but motionless. She would freeze, and then time would telescope, and she would feel not-real, but also intensely real, and like nothing mattered, and also like everything mattered, and like she didn't care about it, but she really did. She would freeze, but underneath the frozen ice was panic, her heart racing, her mind racing, a noodly feeling in her arms and legs like she might pass out, and yet a curious detachment, an observance of this about-to-pass-out-ness. It has been happening daily, for months. Sitting in class, taking a test, talking with friends, having fun. There's no trigger, no warning. Just, suddenly, everything is not-real, and she feels very far away from herself, and at the same time completely at the mercy of her body, her heart hammering at her to pay attention, to realize this feeling of nothing being real is actually real.

She finds herself in the nurse's office, unable to explain what is going on. It feels impossible to say that she feels as though nothing is real, that everything is made up, because if that were true, then why is everything so horrible? If she's making up the entire world, imagining it in her head, then shouldn't the world be better? Shouldn't it be a better place? Shouldn't she be feeling normal? Shouldn't her parents not be divorcing? Shouldn't I not be sick?

So I tell her about the glass delusion. About the ways in which glass was alluring yet terrifying—how could it be so strong, yet so fragile? How could it be bent to make a cup or a bowl without breaking? How could it look smooth as liquid but actually be solid? How could it keep the world out while allowing us to see what lies beyond the walls? I tell her about the glassmaker, the man who understood better than anyone the powers of glass, the ways in which it could be controlled, the mysteries of its existence, and how, for a time, he believed himself to be made of just such fragile stuff. I told her, for comedic value, about how he believed his butt was made of glass, and how his doctor literally kicked his ass to make him realize he was not a glass person, but an actual person. A person who felt pain.

The glass delusion—standing frozen, barely moving, trapped inside his own imagination—was a way to control the uncontrollable. It was a way to protect himself from vulnerability. From pain. From grief. From sadness.

"I think this is a little bit like what's happening to you right now," I tell her. "You're freezing, and feeling like everything isn't real, because the alternative is to feel how angry and anxious and sad you really are."

At this she collapses in my arms, sobbing, the glass broken.

"Everything is so awful," she says. "And I just feel so scared all the time."

"I know," I say, holding her.

"I'm hurting all the time," she says. And I want to say, "Me too," but this isn't about me, and isn't about my pain.

"I know, I know, I know," I say, instead. "Pain is terrifying. And it feels like if you let it in for even a moment, you'll drown in it. But it's going to be okay. You're going to be okay. We're going to be okay. There's a way through this, we'll get through this."

We hold each other for a long time, both of us crying, both of us letting in the light.

One night Nate takes me aside and asks me if he can ask me a very serious question.

"It's okay if you cry a little bit when you answer," he reassures me, "because I know you cry sometimes when you talk about things you care about a lot."

I tell him I will do my best, and so he takes a deep breath and says, "You know when you first got sick, and you told us about getting the divorce, you said that you had thought about it for a really long time before you made the decision, and that you'd thought about it even more after making the decision, before you finally told us."

"I remember," I say.

"Well," he says, "how long did you think about it? And why did you think about it so long? And why did you decide to do it? Was it to protect us? Or what?"

"Those are good questions. I'm going to have to think about them for a bit, too, before I answer you," I say, laughing, stalling for time. How much information does he really need? What is it that he really wants to know?

I had been frozen in place in my marriage for a very long time, unsure of what to do, afraid that if I moved, everything would shatter. I had been a barrier between my kids and their father's anger and absence, and also a conduit between them, facilitating information, explaining what he'd really meant when he'd said what he'd said, or interpreting tone for them, or providing them with strategies for understanding and communicating with someone who was often difficult for them to understand or communicate with. I had been reflecting back to them a false image of a healthy and functioning relationship, mirroring what I thought they needed to see in order to learn to have healthy and functioning relationships themselves. There was a time when they were young when I thought this was what I needed to do to make everything work, just stay still and do what I could to keep things from breaking. But eventually I realized everything was already broken—and, more than that, that they could clearly see it.

I remember talking with my therapist, back when the realization that divorce was inevitable was still just an awful dread in the pit of my stomach, the kind of terrible truth I recognized as a thing I would have to confront no matter how much I wanted to avoid it. I told her, "I feel as though I've been standing on this window ledge for years now, waiting to jump, and it's been the fear of falling that keeps me from making the leap. But if I'm honest with myself, it's probably equally as much because I know that if I turned around from this ledge and looked through the window, I'd see a room—maybe not big enough for me, or comfortable enough, but warm and safe, or familiar at least. And just knowing that's there, that I could just climb back in there anytime I wanted to, makes it harder to jump, and so I feel like I'm forever just standing here on this ledge, not jumping."

She replied: "Remember, though, that you don't *have* to jump."

And then, while I sat there trying to figure out what other option I could possibly have available to me, she said, "See that room where you can look through the window, that safe, familiar, comfortable room? That room also has a door. You could climb back through the window, walk through the room, open the door, and walk down the stairs, step by step, until you get to the ground."

Finally, I begin to try to answer Nate's questions.

"You're right, I thought about it for a really long time. Because it was a very big decision to make, a really important decision that affected a lot of people, and I didn't want to be hasty or reckless or do anything in a way that would make this already hard thing harder on you guys. But I would rather you see how it's possible to move to a healthier place, even though it hurts, than learn to just stay in a bad situation. And of course I thought about it for a long time because I didn't want to cause either of you any pain or heartache, and knowing that this decision would definitely do that, even if it was the right thing to do in the long run, was really hard to think about."

We both cry as I talk, because we both tend to cry when we talk about things that are important to us, and he hugs me tight once I'm done.

"Well," he says, "for what it's worth, I think you made the right call."

I laugh. "Oh, you do?"

"Yeah," he says. "I mean, I was twelve, and twelve is kind of the age when you realize you're not the center of the world, and that bad things happen. Like, you got really sick, and you guys got divorced. It was like a rite of passage, I guess."

"I'm sorry, Nate," I say. "I wish everything could have stayed the same, that I hadn't gotten sick and that our family didn't have to change, that everything could have just kept going, no rite of passage necessary."

I'm touched by his encouragement, and his candor, but also acutely aware of how he, too, has a tendency toward being glass, toward being still and utterly translucent when scared, toward mirroring a soothing reflection to mask his own anxiety.

"You know, the other reason I thought about everything for a long time," I tell him, "was because it took me a very long time to understand my own feelings. And it was very important to me that I sort through my own feelings of sadness and worry and grief, so that I would have enough room to help you deal with your feelings without you ever having to worry about protecting me from them. I'm glad you feel okay about things right now, but I also want you to know that I understand if you don't feel okay about things. Because you might not, from time to time. And that's normal. That's how it works. And I'm okay with that. You don't need to feel bad or protect me from those feelings."

He nods, hugging me. "Grief is complicated," he says.

For Emi, the way out of being frozen in place, as brittle and fragile as glass, is, neatly, through glass. I arrange for her to begin meeting with a therapist, who helps her learn strategies to cope with her panic attacks and stress, and she and I continue to talk about it as well; but what ultimately helps her fully emerge from her frozen panic is finding a way to capture it through a camera lens.

The summer before she applies to college, she spends a month in Manhattan, taking an intensive summer course in photography, an emerging passion of hers. That month is a new space for both of us: for her, being away from her regular life, from my illness and recovery, from the process of our family reconfiguring itself, from traveling between houses and gradually learning to unfreeze; for me, healing from the procedure I have done in North Carolina to fix the leak, recovering from the effects of the leak itself, beginning, however tentatively, to return to a life outside of my bed.

During her time in New York, she finds a set of novelty sunglasses, the lenses fractured into a repeating series of small glass prisms, and places them over the lens of her camera, shooting through them to create a dazzling, discombobulating, unsettling distortion effect that mirrors her experience of feeling dissociated from reality. She calls these photos her "Anxiety Series," some black and white, some color, all simultaneously confusing and claustrophobic and fascinating. She does the thing that artists do, and takes her very personal experience and transmutes it into something someone else can understand in a visceral, powerful, immediate way. Her use of light is stunning, her subjects intriguing, her perspective and voice compelling. And the act of creating this very personal art is healing in a way she doesn't fully realize until her panic attacks and feelings of being frozen in place, at the mercy of a world both too real and unreal, are gone.

The way out for me is less clear-cut. I can't see my way through to the end point of my recovery, where this part of my life will be a memory. It's like trying to look through a one-way mirror, and only seeing myself reflected back at me. Time, my doctors tell me, is the only data point they have to offer in terms of what will make me heal. Time and luck, both as fragile as glass.

Deep in the brain, hidden in the dark recesses, is a small gland, shaped like a pinecone and about the size of a grain of rice. It's the only part of the brain that stands alone, unpaired: In the midst of the mirror-image left and right hemispheres, tucked into the center where the two halves of the thalamus meet, the pineal gland sits, singular. It, like the rest of the brain, is bathed in cerebrospinal fluid; in the case of the pineal gland, this is supplied to it by the nearby third ventricle. Its small size belies its importance: It is an endocrine organ, responsible for governing our sleep patterns and circadian rhythms, a feat it accomplishes by producing melatonin. The timing and amount of melatonin it produces is triggered by cycles of darkness, when it produces more, and light, when it produces less. And so in that sense it shouldn't be surprising to learn that the pineal gland, sequestered though it might be in the darkest, deepest center of the brain, as far as possible away from light, is actually light-sensitive, a deep-brain nonvisual photoreceptor. Our retinas perceive light, and pass this information along to a part of the hypothalamus called the suprachiasmatic nucleus, which relays this information to another group of neurons in the hypothalamus called the paraventricular nucleus, which relays this information to the spinal cord and superior cervical ganglion, which, finally, relays this information to the pineal gland. Well before this process was understood, however, the pineal gland was a subject of intrigue for anatomists, philosophers, and mystics alike. Descartes called the pineal gland "the seat of the soul"; the nineteenth-century Russian occultist Helena Blavatsky suggested a connection between the pineal gland and the Hindu concept of the all-seeing "third eye," the Ajna chakra. Taoists call this area, where the pineal and pituitary glands are located, "the crystal palace."

A palace made of glass.

This crystal palace in the brain is a fragile information system, sending and interpreting signals, responding and regulating, all of it built and functioning without the awareness of the mind. In fact, the work of the brain goes on entirely without the mind, which is its own glass palace, its own hall of mirrors, alternately a telescope, a magnifying glass, a portal, a boundary, a microscope, a prism of focus, a fibrous cable of information, a thin pane through which to view the world.

The fragile work of illness and recovery, the fracturing of the crystal palace in my brain, and its self-repair, reminds me of the dual nature of glass, the strength and clarity of it, the breakable nature of it. The way that glass is neither pure liquid nor pure solid, but rather exists someplace between those two states.

This breakdown of my marriage, this sudden and mysterious and debilitating illness, is my own version of the glassmaker's kick in the butt—the realization of my own pain, the undeniable nature of my very real physical pain, the legitimizing of my emotional pain—shattering the delusion that pain is a thing from which I can protect myself or anyone else. My being frozen in place, as still and smooth as glass, doesn't save me from being shattered, just traps me in perpetual fear of shattering. And so, like Emi with her photographs, like Nate with his questions and clarity, like the glassmaker finally being freed, I must allow myself to move. To feel. To remind myself that it's okay to cry a little when I talk about it. To inhabit the place where I am both liquid and solid, fluid and in stasis, fixed and in the process of becoming, reflecting, refracting, and revealing this new self I am just now beginning to understand.

27

January 2016

With its low buildings and valet staff on hand as soon as we pull up the day of my tests, Duke University Hospital strikes me as resembling the hotels surrounding it, albeit with less signage about its daily rates. Just inside the entrance, hanging over the entryway to the main lobby, is a curved plexiglass banner of sorts that reads "Welcome to the Duke Experience." The Duke Experience sounds less like a way to describe a hospital visit than it does the name of a competitive college a cappella show choir, and it amuses me to imagine the medical professionals, in their off-hours, working to tighten their harmonies and choreo for Nationals.

It's a surprisingly straightforward path to the radiology department, no elevators or endless hallways to negotiate, just straight through the lobby with its leafy plants and shiny piano, and then a left at the elevator bank, and then another left, and there we are at the check-in desk, where friendly administrators tell me in the kindest way possible that my post-divorce COBRA insurance hasn't kicked in yet, and promise to hold off on billing me for just a bit, but make me sign a bunch of pages on a clipboard anyway saying that I'll be responsible for the $25,000 bill if the insurance company doesn't come through. And then I sit in the nubby tan-orange waiting area chairs, as slumped down as possible, to be as flat as possible, until my name is called and another friendly person takes me back to a room where I change into a maxi dress of a hospital gown and then, thankfully, sit in a special chair, just for people like me, which reclines to the point of almost full horizontal.

When the physician assistant comes in, he says, "No no, don't sit up," and finds a way to hover over me in a non-looming, non-awkward manner, and asks me all the same questions I've been asked for months and months now. Except this time, as I answer, he nods his head in recognition, and he doesn't look at me with skepticism, and he seems to accept everything I say as utterly normal and not surprising in the least, and instead of this coming off as his being unimpressed I see he is merely recognizing that all of these things that I'm describing, which appeared so exotic and nonsensical and difficult to believe to the other medical professionals I've seen, are the same symptoms described to him by literally every patient who comes here.

"So this is normal," I say, and he says, "We see it all the time." And when I ask why it's so invisible to all these other doctors—doctors at important places, world-renowned centers of academia, hospitals with peerless research facilities—he explains that this is like a sub-specialty of a sub-specialty of a sub-specialty, and that even when papers are published about it, those journals go to generalists who first of all may not ever read the journals (I nod my head, remembering the unread towers of the *American Journal of Ophthalmology* that became a part of the furniture when Gil and I were married), and second of all may only have time to even skim just the most important articles in their own field, and so they'll never read about this, and probably only rarely encounter it, if ever. And so the things that seem normal to everyone in this place are strange and unfamiliar to nearly everyone outside it—and, because these things are patient-reported symptoms, eminently doubtable. "We could publish the cure for cancer in there," he says, "and nobody would know about it."

He explains today's tests—how they'll do a lumbar puncture and take a baseline pressure reading, even though opening pressure doesn't really signify anything clinically one way or the other, and then inject radiopaque dye and put me in a CT scanner to see if they are able to see the leak in action. "And if you don't?" I ask. "Well, the doctor will talk to you about that," he says. "But probably we'll patch you up anyway. To be honest, most of the time the leaks don't show. If they do, then we know exactly where the leak is and we can be more precise about where we do the patching. But if they don't, we can still patch you."

After all the questions are done, he leaves, and I take a lorazepam to help with anxiety and claustrophobia, though I've been assured that I won't have to go too deep into the CT scanner or be there for too long, and I consider adjusting the mechanical chair to sit myself up more before the doctor comes in to talk to me, because isn't this taking it a little too far, lying down so flat, isn't this a little self-indulgent, I'm not that bad, and isn't giving in making it worse?

Dr. Kranz comes in, baby-faced and tall, and I feel bad making him hover over me as I lie flat, but he, too, seems to accept this as normal and not rude at all, and again I realize I'm in a different place here, a place where everyone understands the importance of being flat, where no one thinks it self-indulgent for a person to lie back in an impression of someone who is relaxing. He asks many of the same questions, and goes over the procedure in a little more depth, and confirms for me that this is, indeed, real, and that from my symptoms, I am indeed experiencing spontaneous intracranial hypotension, and that there are routine procedures here that can help.

In the room for the procedure, I'm placed on my side and I'm glad for the lorazepam I took earlier as a needle is stuck in my back. The physician assistant and the nurses have a running banter I understand to have been honed over the heads of hundreds of other patients, like me, lying on their sides and terrified. The jokes put me at ease, and their easiness puts me at ease, and I find myself laughing even when they're telling me, "Be still and try not to laugh," and then the fluid is injected and although at first I feel an uncomfortable twang and then a nerve-twinging pressure, within minutes I feel a blissful buoyancy and fullness in my head. "Oh, I feel my brain working again," I say, as they start to roll me onto my back and have me start moving from side to side and doing bridge pose and something they call "log rolling," in which I am the log being rolled, and otherwise jiggering the fluid around so that it moves along my spine, the better to light everything up once I'm in the scanner. "Well, you've got some fluid in there now," they say, and remark that that's another sign that this really is a CSF leak, the fact that I feel so much better with this extra fluid pumped into the CSF space, making my brain float again after so many months without a cushion. I lie there, only slightly panicking and claustrophobic as I slide into the CT scanner up to my neck, and hope the images show something, anything, so that tomorrow the doctors will be able to know exactly where to place the patch, to fix this thing, to end this madness.

That night, in the hotel, my sister brings in food, and a friend I've only known from the internet comes to meet me in person, and, buoyed by a floaty brain from the bolus of fluid injected earlier, which has not yet had a chance to fully seep out, I sit up while I eat dinner, for the first time in months, stay up talking and making jokes, for the first time in months, sit up on the couch instead of lying down and follow the thread of a conversation for more than an hour, for the first time in months. The fog lifts, briefly, and, for the first time in months, I feel almost normal.

The next morning, before returning to the hospital for the procedure that will hopefully fix me, I get a phone call from the therapist's office where I've been trying to set up an appointment for Emi, so she can talk with someone besides me about the stress and dissociation of dealing with a sick mom, divorcing parents. The normalcy I felt the night before has drained away, and my brain is back to its fuzzy functionality. "What is your daughter's birth date?" the receptionist asks me, and I pause for an embarrassingly long time. *You know this*, I tell myself, and I know that this is true—I can *feel* when Emi's birthday is, I can feel the feeling of what the words are that might contain that information, I have a sense of what the numbers would feel like to say out loud. It is there, somewhere, in my brain. But I can't remember. I can't say it out loud. It stays formless inside me, a mere suspicion, a hunch, while the receptionist repeats "Ma'am?" and I say, "Sorry, one moment," stalling for time. I'm just about to ask my sister if she might remember when Emi's birthday is, when I hear myself beginning to say "June?" And then I remember: "June 3, 1999, six-three-nine-nine." I say it both ways, words and numbers, and somehow that unlocks the door to the other fact-based answers I must give—our address, a date and time that works for me to bring her in—and I am able to finish the phone call successfully.

I remember to say goodbye. I remember to tap the red phone icon to hang up. *After today*, I think, as I get ready to go to the hospital, *a conversation like this might be a thing of the past. After today, I might be better.*

But at the hospital, my hopes are dashed when Dr. Kranz returns, pulling up a chair beside the recliner where I, too, have returned, his baby-face forehead now creased with concern, and tells me he was not able to visualize the leak. I am in the 50 percent or so of people for whom the leak site is not observed on CT myelogram. It is all I can do to keep myself from crying. This is my worst-case scenario: that they are unable to find the leak and thus unable to treat me. That I will be like this forever.

"Are there stronger tests, finer tests?" I ask, and he says, "Yes, we could do an MRI myelogram—although of those patients who go on to have that done, only 20 percent have a positive result or identifiable leak." *So that's it*, I think, *it's over*, and I struggle to keep my face calm, my voice even, as I ask, "So now what?"

"Now," he says, surprising me, "we treat you."

Even though they can't see the exact location of the leak, he tells me that in his experience, most patients with symptoms like mine are leaking from somewhere in their thoracic spine, the upper and middle back area that extends from the base of the neck to just a few inches below the shoulder blades. So what they'll do today is patch me there—inject my own blood into the epidural space along my spine between my shoulder blades, and also several other places along my spine, so as to seal the dura, creating a kind of Band-Aid of blood to clot over any torn places. "If we knew exactly where the leak was, we'd do a more targeted patch, with a mixture of blood and fibrin—an insoluble protein that impedes blood flow—right in the leak spot. But since we don't, we can patch more generally in that area, just using blood."

"So you can treat me," I say, and he nods. "Even though you can't find the leak."

He nods again. "I don't have to see the leak to know that you're leaking."

Again I am in the procedure room, again with the friendly nurses making jokes over my head. This time I am instructed to lie on my stomach, a blood pressure cuff on one arm, an IV in the other, so they'll be able to access my IV for blood as the doctor needs it to inject into my back. This time I get a mixture of fentanyl and Versed (midazolam), and it feels like nothing. I don't think it's working at all, until I find myself struggling to get comfortable, facedown on the table, and hear myself saying too loudly that I wished there were some kind of hole for my face. "Does anyone know, is there, like, some kind of face-hole, does anyone have a hole I could put my face in?" I ask, and everyone laughs, and then to my amazement someone does indeed produce a hole I could put my face in: some kind of massage-table contraption thing one of the comedian nurses brings over and helps me settle my face into. I can't stop laughing at the coincidence of my needing a face-hole and them happening to have one handy, and I realize as I'm slid into the CT scanner feet-first that the medication must be working.

They inject my back with lidocaine—lots of lidocaine. I'd warned them of my redheaded need for more pain medication, and yet it still surprises them that I'm able to feel things that by all accounts I should have been numbed to several injections before. But finally my back is anesthetized enough to allow the doctor to introduce needles into my spine without my feeling every part of it.

Later, Dr. Kranz would show me a video of a straightforward procedure like mine, a series of still photos from the CT scanner strung together into a stop-motion movie, captured with a foot pedal he'd tapped while his hands busied themselves with the work of placing needles in such a way that they were able to deliver an injection of the patient's own blood to the space around the spinal cord without piercing anything that shouldn't be pierced. "This is the spinal column, like a stack of marshmallows," he indicated, pointing to a row of white blobs on the screen. In the next frame, a close-up of the spine at the location of a suspected leak, he pointed out a bony arch with little gaps in it. "Those gaps are where we want to go," ideally poking the needle into a gray area just above where the CSF and spinal cord are contained by the dura. Then a flash of white appeared on-screen: contrast dye, to visualize where the blood would be injected, to make sure it would be going into the place it's supposed to go, coating the dura rather than being injected directly into the spinal fluid. After that, the blood was injected, and the stop-motion movie captured the way it spread along and around the dura, sealing it up with blood that would, eventually, clot and plug up any holes.

This was something I would see only later, though, long after my procedure was done. From my vantage point during the procedure, with my face in the face-hole, I have only a vague sense of what's happening at the moment, which, thanks to the fentanyl and Versed, is fine with me. I lie facedown on the table, halfway in the CT scanner, my face in the face-hole, one arm up near my left ear with a blood pressure cuff squeezing it every few minutes, the other arm up near my right ear with an IV in it for delivering the pain meds and accessing my vein for blood to use in the blood patch. Dr. Kranz explains what he's doing as he does it, and tells me each time he places a needle. I'm alert enough to hear the difference in his tone when he's speaking to me versus speaking to the nurses and physician assistant, when he's noting something for my benefit or noting something for theirs. I can't feel the needles, but each time, once they're in and he begins injecting the blood, I feel the familiar nerve-twinging sensation of pressure building in my spine, and again have to answer the question of how much pressure is too much. It's impossible to know. It's an uncomfortable feeling, a feeling of wrongness, that something is absolutely not right, and so immediately I want to say "too much," but then I worry that my "too much" might still be not enough, so I try to wait until the last possible moment of feeling that kind of twangy, jangly, reflexy feeling, like when the doctor has you dangle your leg and hits just below your kneecap to induce a kick, except that it's that feeling on the inside of your back, along your spine, between your shoulder blades, and then between your lower ribs, and then between your kidneys, and then between your hips.

Eventually I say "too much" in each spot, and I hear the doctor note for himself and his assistants and for me, too, how my blood is spreading, how he can see it coating the dura well in each of the areas he's injected. And then, miraculously, it's over: My blood has been injected in the right places, has spread the way he needs it to spread. Now my back is swabbed with something cold, the blood pressure cuff removed, the face-hole returned to its mysterious hiding place. The doctor says all has gone well, that he'll check in with me in recovery in a bit. Nurses help me roll over to lie on my back, move me to a gurney that transports me to a recovery room. Everything is ceiling and upside-down faces for a while as I float in my fentanyl haze.

Later I would read the medical account of the procedure, accessible through the patient portal online. It's how I discovered my extra, rudimentary set of ribs.

The patient was placed in the prone position on the CT table, and a scout image was obtained for localization purposes. The patient's IV was accessed, and 5 mL of blood was wasted. Additional blood was collected in multiple syringes under sterile fashion. Interlaminar epidural blood patches were placed using

CT fluoroscopic guidance and 3.5" 22-gauge spinal needles at the levels listed below. Prior to each injection, a small amount of Isovue-M 200 contrast was injected to confirm epidural, extravascular location. Note that there is transitional anatomy, with 13 pairs of ribs, with the inferior most level representing rudimentary ribs. For the purposes of this dictation, the level of the rudimentary ribs will be designated as L1.

T9-10 (left posterior oblique interlaminar approach, 4 mL autologous blood injected)

L1-2 (left posterior oblique interlaminar approach, 8 mL autologous blood injected)

T4-5 (left posterior oblique interlaminar approach, 3 mL autologous blood injected)

L4-5 (left posterior oblique interlaminar approach, 5 mL autologous blood injected)

The needles were removed. The patient tolerated the procedure well without complication. She was taken to the recovery room in good condition.

Estimated blood loss: Negligible. Patient was given contact information and instructions for follow-up.

Impression: Successful epidural blood patches at a total of 4 levels in the thoracic and lumbar spine, as above.

My version of the story has a face-hole and anxiety and nerve-twinging pressure. The medical notes version has clinical language, secret ribs, and exact anatomical locations.

Both of these stories are true.

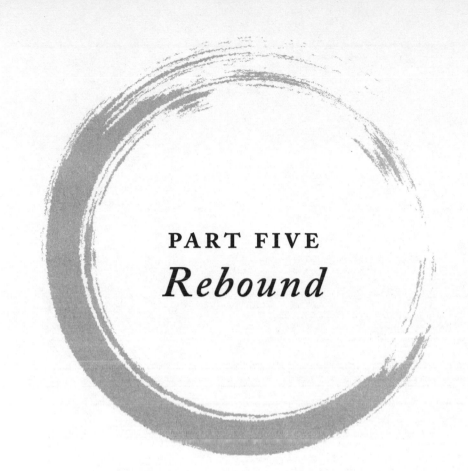

PART FIVE

Rebound

28

In the hospital, I lie flat on a bed in the recovery area. I'm given crackers, a drink. I talk with my sister, groggy, in a haze, from drugs this time rather than the normal haze of my leaky brain. Dr. Kranz comes in and leans over me, talking about the procedure he just performed, talking about my prognosis, about restrictions on lifting, bending, walking, sex.

I may experience an increase in intracranial pressure, he tells me. My body has been overproducing cerebrospinal fluid to compensate for the leak; now that the leak has been patched—for the moment, at least—it may take some time for my body to realize it, to lower production to more normal levels. This may cause what's called rebound intracranial hypertension: too much cerebrospinal fluid instead of too little. This usually takes the form of a headache in the front of the head, and may also be accompanied by blurry vision, nausea, vomiting. I think back to the way I felt after my first blood patch, the way my head felt like it might explode, the headaches all over the front of my face. I have been through this before. He tells me that I should try to avoid lying completely flat, try to prop my pillows up to give myself about a thirty-degree slope to lie on—not sitting up, which can stress the dura, and not lying down, which can increase my intracranial pressure; but rather some sweet spot in between. This will help with the rebound headaches, he tells me.

He writes me a prescription for pain medication, and for something to treat nausea, and for something called Diamox, but he folds that paper in half before he gives it to me. "Do not fill this prescription without talking to me first," he says. "This is for 'in case of emergency.'" He will call me tomorrow and the next day to check in; if my rebound symptoms are unbearable, we will consider the Diamox—but he'd rather avoid it, if we can. Diamox, also known as acetazolamide, is a diuretic, which can help with the excess fluid; but it's a serious medication that decreases CSF production and has its own unpleasant side effects. He'd like to see if we can give my body a chance to adapt and readjust on its own before we take that route. And since only my own blood was used in the patching of my dura, and not fibrin sealant or some other biologically based glue, the overall patch itself is a little flexible, and thus may more easily weather the flux of increased fluid. The other option in the case of rebound intracranial hypertension, he tells me, besides just time and waiting things out or taking Diamox, is coming back to the hospital and having my cerebrospinal fluid drained a little, to relieve the pressure. "Let's go with the healing powers of the passage of time," I say, and he agrees that that's a good conservative approach to start with.

"So, what now?" I ask, and he understands I mean to ask the question in the larger sense.

"Now?" he says. "Now we wait."

It may take two months for me to fully heal from the procedure I've just had, and then another two to three months to tell whether or not I might still be leaking. Even with the patching, I could have a very slow, subtle leak, whose symptoms could very easily be confused with the kind of symptoms that are normal during recovery—headaches that get worse as the day goes on, stamina that fades, the need to lie down, pain that improves upon lying down. I could develop a new leak, if my cerebrospinal fluid pressure doesn't settle, if the patch on my torn dura isn't able to keep it shut during the surge. It's just going to take time to know what's happening, whether I'm healing or still leaking, and he tells me it's not unusual for patients to return two, three, even five or six times, for repeat procedures.

"What about one time, no repeat procedures?" I ask, and he smiles. "There's always that chance," he says. "You could get lucky."

The absolute best-case scenario—if I truly am lucky and everything goes perfectly—is that I spend a few days in the hotel, return home, recover over the next few months with no recurrence of the leak, and never have to come back.

"And if all that goes according to plan, in the absolute best-case scenario, how long until I'm back to normal? In my brain, I mean," I ask, and he tells me it'll probably take about a year to get back to baseline.

A year seems like a long time. Longer than the amount of time I've dealt with the pain of this leak, though that seems infinite and thus impossible to calculate. I have the urge to take this deadline as a challenge, to not only attempt the best-case scenario recovery, but to do it faster than anyone expects, to do it better, to win. This impulse is probably an artifact of the Versed and fentanyl euphoria that's still affecting me, this curious feeling of motivation instead of dauntedness. But for the moment, as I lie there in the recovery bed, my blood clotting around my spine like a living Band-Aid, making the length of it heavy, solid, detectable, and sensate to me in a way it has never been before, I feel as lifted up as I am weighted down.

Eventually I am returned to my clothes, which have never seemed so impossible to put on, and wheeled to the entrance of the hospital, where I wait for my sister to pull up her car. My head is already full-feeling, packed tight with drugs and fluid and information: I am not to lift anything heavier than a gallon of milk for the first month or so, then nothing heavier than fifteen to twenty pounds; I am not to bend or twist, I must lower myself down with my knees, I must turn my whole body and not crane my neck or twist my spine; I should sleep propped up with pillows; I should try to walk around a little when I can, as tolerated, with the guideline of X minutes of upright time equaling X minutes of lying down time; I should try to avoid caffeine and sodium, both of which can raise intracranial pressure.

When my sister arrives, I stand up from the wheelchair and walk for the first time since going in to my procedure. Suddenly the gravity is different on this planet. I move so slowly, and my back feels so tight. We both laugh as I attempt to walk through the hospital's massive revolving door: It's a rotating chamber, wide enough to fit a gurney or several wheelchairs at once, moving so slowly as to be nearly imperceptible, and yet I can barely shuffle fast enough to get through it. I walk so slowly that the door catches up with me, pushing me out into the world, my discharge papers and prescriptions in hand, the one "in case of emergency" prescription still folded, placed for safekeeping in a zippered pocket of my purse, which is too heavy for me to carry.

I lie down in the passenger seat, as reclined as possible, and Jessie drives us back to the hotel. The walk from the car to our room takes hours, it seems. I can't carry anything, and Jessie goes back and forth several times, ferrying things between the car and the room, in the time it takes me to baby-step my way there just once. Once I'm installed in the hotel bed, propped up on pillows, Jessie leaves to fill the prescriptions. The pain medication from the morning's procedure is wearing off, and Tylenol is not helping. She calls me from the pharmacy: evidently my COBRA insurance has not kicked in, and the medication must be bought at full cost. I authorize her to buy it anyway, and she does, bringing me home Norco (a combination of acetaminophen and hydrocdone, for the pain) and Zofran (also known as ondansetron, for the nausea), along with low-sodium snacks and foods for me to eat when I can.

The Norco sends me into a lovey, overly affectionate daze— Jessie wisely takes my phone away from me after I begin texting everyone I know, telling them that I love them and that they're the best, and laughs when I answer her question of how the medication is affecting me by telling her, "You know the feeling you feel, like, *right* after you have sex? *That's* what this feels like!"—but the effects only last for so long. The more I take it, the less good I feel, and eventually taking it makes me feel bad, causing me anxiety and paranoia, and so I stop and revert to plain old Tylenol, taking the Norco only when I can't take the pain any longer.

By the next afternoon, when Dr. Kranz calls me to follow up, I am in full-blown rebound high pressure. My head feels like a pain-filled balloon attached to an aching lead pipe, I am nauseated from the pressure and pain, my eyes hurt, everything hurts. He reminds me to find that sweet spot, that thirty-degree angle of uprightness in bed that can help me tolerate the pressure and pain. He still says to hold off on the Diamox, to not fill that prescription yet, to try to keep managing things without. This may be the worst of it, he says, and perhaps I can ride it out until my body starts to adjust. He says he'll call back the next day to see how I'm doing, reminds me to take the Zofran to deal with the nausea, to avoid caffeine and sodium.

I'm cleared to take a shower by this point, but I can't lift my arms over my head to take off my shirt. I try to put my hair in a ponytail, but even that is excruciating. It takes several attempts, and I have to take breaks during each try. The space between my shoulder blades is particularly heavy, and reaching my arms up sets it on fire. I return to the bed and take more medicine and my sister brings me food and I try to will my body to adjust, to stop ballooning my head with fluid, to stop flooding that fluid along my spine and aggravating the site of the leak.

Dr. Kranz had said that even though they couldn't visualize the leak through imaging, it was likely that it was in my thoracic spine, somewhere between my shoulder blades, and I feel it there now, the burning, the pressure. An ice pack helps; being slightly propped up instead of flat helps. My dura is so tight, with my blood clotted and coiled around it, that I have instant feedback about what strains it: my chin down as I look at my phone, my posture slumped when I stand up. These things trigger a jolt of pain, and I am reminded to keep my chin up, or at least neutral, to stand with my back straight.

The drive back to Philadelphia is long and bumpy, despite the pain meds. We listen to podcasts and talk a little; I am uncomfortable and in pain, worried that every jolt will undo the procedure I had done, drifty with the medication, grateful for my sister's patience and help. Once home, every step is a challenge. I'd forgotten the existence of stairs in my house, had never before considered them a provocation. But now they are an unclimbable mountain. Jessie helps me inside, carrying my bags upstairs for me, and I collapse on the couch on the first floor. I will sleep there. It will take me another day before I can make the climb to my bedroom, at the top of Mount Everest, the third floor.

These are the practicalities of recovery:

A wedge-shaped pillow, a giant thirty-degree foam triangle, for sleeping and existing in bed.

A grabber stick, with a handle to squeeze and pinchers to grasp, so that I can pick things up without bending.

A giant cooler near my bed with bottles of water and flavored drinks, ice.

A small table within arm's reach, for all my medicines and chargers and things I might need to get without getting up to get them.

Ice turbans, ice packs that wrap around my head and Velcro into place, encasing my skull in cold and distracting from the ever-present high-pressure headache.

Dandelion leaf tea, a leaker-group standby, recommended for post-patching rebound high pressure, to be drunk in the afternoons, when the headache is at its worst.

Eventually, when I can move around, when I can do chores: a long scooper for the litter boxes, a tall-handled dustpan for the broom.

Some of these things—the cooler, the table—are the same things I used before recovering, when I was leaking. But life post-procedure is the opposite of leak life: All the things that used to help ameliorate my pain—caffeine, salt, lying flat—now exacerbate it. Now I drink water, now I pine for Diet Coke and Doritos, now I sleep on the uncomfortable wedge pillow to alleviate pressure. Sitting—merely sitting like a human—is the worst: It stresses my dura and results in a near-instantaneous headache that can take hours to resolve.

Dr. Kranz advised me to think of this recovery time in days, not hours; in weeks, not days; to gauge my progress in months, not weeks. My brain is still foggy, squeezed by so much cerebrospinal fluid, which my body is still overproducing to compensate for the leak it doesn't yet realize has been fixed, however temporarily. Recovering will take time.

When the kids come back home, I try to explain to them how I am in opposite-world now, how being upright is still exhausting at this point, but being flat is worse, how everything that helped with the leak hurts it now. I tell them to imagine a garden hose, like the one we have out back on the patio. "Imagine there's a hole somewhere along the hose, and so when you turn on the water, it kind of just trickles out, because of how the water is leaking through the hole somewhere along the way. And so you turn the water up full blast, just to get something close to regular water pressure coming out of the end of the hose. Now imagine you leave the water running like that while you patch up the hole, put a piece of duct tape over it or whatever. What happens to the water coming out of the hose once you fix that hole? It shoots out at full pressure, now that there's no hole to drain any water away. That's what's happening right now with my cerebrospinal fluid," I tell them. "My brain doesn't realize yet that the hole is patched, and it's still sending that water out full blast, it hasn't yet realized it can turn the faucet back to normal. That part is going to take some time, and that's why I have a different kind of headache now."

They help me through this, step up with the chores and cat duties, abide my funny-looking ice-pack turban, my still-foggy brain, my still-present pain. Gradually, as my spine begins to stop feeling like it's made of solid lead, I start to increase my upright time. I walk around the house, wiping counters, doing laundry, sorting mail, making dinner. I walk outside for five minutes, ten minutes, twenty. I wear my ice pack around my head in the afternoons, I drink dandelion tea.

These are the impracticalities of recovery:

The way it happens in real time, and the way real time is slow and inexorable.

The way it happens nonlinearly, despite my moving through time on a linear trajectory.

Progress seems to erase itself even as it is happening, and I am only able to understand a sense of momentum, of change, if I look at the points I have plotted along the way as a shape that unfolds over time, without getting stuck in those individual moments that seem to be permanently folded.

The way it is impossible to gauge, no signposts, no red flags other than the new headache slowly, imperceptibly becoming the old headache, the post-patching headache becoming the leak headache.

The way it is impossible to trust. Even if the seal holds, even if my body gradually adjusts, even if my brain returns to making a normal amount of cerebrospinal fluid, and even if my dura withstands the daily ebb and flow of its production, there is no guarantee that this once-torn place will not rip through. I have hemmed a skirt, I have mended tears in the knees of pants, I have knitted up sweaters that have unraveled; I understand the fragility of the sewn-up thing, the new tentativity at the site of the repair. I know the chance exists that this mended spot will always be a tender place.

The way it is a mystery, the path back to baseline health as unfathomable and beyond my control as the journey into illness. I must wait for my choroid plexus to slow the production of fluid, I must wait as my dura knits itself back together beneath the protective layer of my own clotted blood, which over time dissolves away, leaving the torn spot bare. I must wait as my brain re-rights itself, learns what it's like to float again, stretches the places cramped from months of pain, of sinking. All of this mystery is a grand mystery I myself cannot solve, and cannot hurry.

The way it means relearning, and the way it means forgetting.

Two weeks after my procedure, I leave my bedroom for the first time since being home. I find clothes that are easy to put on, as my arms are still sore, as that spot between my shoulder blades flares with pain and heaviness when I raise them. Emi helps me put on my socks, my winter boots, as I must not bend and cannot reach to do either without bending. It is the end of January, and outside the world is snow and ice, and so we both must bundle up, puffy winter coats, winding scarves, thick hats, warm gloves. Today is her first appointment with a therapist, just a few blocks from our house, and I promised I would take her. My purse is still too heavy for me to carry, so she carries it for me. The sky is gray, but the snow is bright, pocked by patches of ice slicks. Walking for any length of time is still new, being upright is still new—all of this is new, her seeing a therapist, me being in recovery—and so we take our time, going slowly in the searing wind, moving carefully, aware that with each footstep we face the possibility of slipping, of danger. We hold each other as we make our way together across the treacherous city sidewalks, and she reminds me to take my time, to go slow. She holds my hand. She makes sure I'm okay. Together, we make our way across the ice.

Traumatized people are left with an experience of "singularity" that creates a divide between their experience and the consensual reality of others. Part of what makes it traumatic is the lack of communication that is possible about it. "The worlds of traumatized persons are fundamentally incommensurable with those of others," Robert Stolorow writes. Trauma creates a "deep chasm in which an anguished sense of estrangement and solitude takes form."

—Mark Epstein, *The Trauma of Everyday Life*

29

I am an unreliable narrator.

If my illness was about telling my story to my doctors and myself, trying to explain it to myself, my recovery is about telling it to other people, trying to explain it to everyone else.

How are you? What have you been up to? What happened?

These are normal questions, everyday questions, but attempting to answer them seems impossible. At first because any possible answer seems too big—too sprawling and specific, too filled with details that a part of me understands are unnecessary to the asker, who likely doesn't really want to know them.

And then because my brain isn't good yet at sorting through details, understanding perspective, knowing what's important and what's not. I still walk into stores and freeze, unable to parse competing amounts of information: the colors, the lights, the sounds, the aisles, the people, the products, the process. Everything dazzles, everything shouts at me at the exact same volume, everything persists with the same emphasis, the same importance, and I feel myself becoming heavy, pulling down the way I used to feel my brain pulling down, aching itself into me, unable to fight gravity any longer. My thoughts, when I have to speak them, are like that, too. My ability to gauge the appropriateness of shareable information is still unrefined, and every conversation I have is a test, both for myself and for the listener as I pause, weigh, evaluate, think. Attempt to speak. Say too little. Say too much.

And then of course because my story is so odd. I coughed one day, and then my brain stopped working? I spent nine months staring at the ceiling? Oh, and also, during that time when my brain didn't work and I was stuck in bed, I got divorced? How does that even happen?

"What happened?" is the hardest question to answer. It should be the easiest, because there are facts, simple facts, and I can tell people those facts, and those facts are the actual, literal definition of what happened, which is what people are asking me. But it's hard to know where to start, or how many facts to tell, or which ones, and sometimes when I pause too long, people fill in the blanks for me. They look stricken, assuming I'm about to tell them I have cancer, or that my husband died, or that my parents died, or that my children are sick. I see them brace themselves for the worst, and I rush to reassure them, "No, no, I'm fine, everyone's fine, I mean, I got divorced, but it's fine, I'm fine, the kids are okay, we're fine."

Sometimes I say, "I was sick, but I'm better now."

Sometimes I say, "You know that thing that covers your brain and spinal cord?"

Once, while I was still dealing with the leak, I told a friend the truth about what happened. I'd forgotten she had crippling phobias of all things medical, of all things in general, and I told her how I'd coughed and torn my dura and had my cerebrospinal fluid leak out. I saw her visibly pale as my strange sentence of facts went on and on and on, her eyes widening, her body subtly moving itself away from mine, as if I might be contagious. "You got this from coughing?" she asked. I nodded. "Can *anyone* get this from coughing?" she asked. I nodded. "And you're getting divorced?" she asked. I nodded. I was the terrifying Ghost of Christmas Future, a living public service announcement, an After-School Special, a horrible warning, a cautionary tale: *This could happen to you!*

I haven't learned yet, or maybe never properly understood, how to modulate my grief (Is this grief? Is that what healing is?), how to smooth the edges of my rawness so as not to cut too sharply into the comfort of others. It is as though I can hear everyone singing, but my voice struggles to find the key, to fit the proper register, to blend. A writer friend told me, after the death of her child, that being in the world again she felt like the only person who understood that everyone, everywhere, is walking on a tightrope while believing themselves to be on solid ground. She walked so carefully, so gingerly, so slowly, while everyone else strode with purpose, oblivious to the possibility of falling. Her very presence unnerved those who didn't want to believe things could be so precarious. I understood her then; I understand her more now.

It's strange to be in the world again, upright for hours at a time, strange to be a person who stands up and walks around and runs errands, albeit slowly, and is only in bed 60 percent instead of 90 percent of the day. I'm not sure how to be that person yet, and it's strange to venture outside the world of my bed, my room, my house. I walk slowly, and struggle with the pain of my self in recovery—the high-pressure headache, the "off"-ness I feel when I've been upright for too long. It takes focus to walk my therapeutic twenty-minute slow walks around the blocks near my house, and I feel a little bit like an impostor, or at least like a tourist, or at least like a person visiting a place they lived a long time ago and moved away from, who remembers some things but has forgotten others, or who has been away for so long the landscape has changed and all they can see are the differences: new construction where a church used to be, the old restaurant replaced by a new one, with the attendant sense of carrying around with them the person they used to be when they lived there. And yet I still live here, I have lived here, I didn't move away, I never left. It's still all new.

On one of these walks, passing by a place that when I got sick was a neighborhood bar but is now a Korean fusion restaurant, I run into a friend, who stops me on the sidewalk by saying, "Oh my god! I haven't seen you in forever! How are you? What have you been up to? Have you been working on another book?"

I don't have words, and I pause too long, and I see her panic with concern for me, but I can't begin to answer. I feel like I'm visiting from another planet, and trying to explain what I've been up to is like trying to explain how to breathe air in a place with no oxygen. I have to explain the rocket, the liftoff, the journey, the suit, the apparatus, the lonely planet, the trip home. Working on another book seems just as foreign and unlikely an endeavor. Merely answering the question seems as foreign and unlikely an endeavor.

Finally, I say something, because she is hugging me, saying, "Oh god, are you okay?" And I tell her I'm fine, I'm fine, I was sick, but I'm fine, and I'm divorced now, but I'm fine, and the kids are fine, and we're all fine, and I'm lucky, but we're fine.

"What happened?" she asks, and even though she has a friend standing there with her, a stranger I'm sure doesn't want to know what happened, this friend seems to genuinely want to know my answer, or my demeanor is worrying enough to demand an explanation, and so I begin to tell her—the flu, the cough, the strange headache, the diagnosis, the divorce, the nine months of pain, of waiting, of things falling apart, of worry, of not writing or thinking or doing much more than the basics of lying down and trying to be present for my kids, even though I was like a ghost of myself. I explain it to her, not the full story, because I don't know how to begin to tell it then, but the facts of it, as I can remember them, and I try to communicate to her the strangeness of it, then and now, and how even standing there talking to her is a strangeness, because of how I'm standing instead of lying down, and how my head still isn't used to standing, and how my brain is still recovering from all those months of bruising, and how I don't know yet whether or not the leak is fixed, it's been two months, almost three months since I was patched, and I won't know for maybe six months if I'm really okay, whether the leak is truly repaired, and the whole time I'm telling her this, I'm thinking *What is her name?*—this person I've known for roughly sixteen years, who lives blocks away from me, whose kids are the same age as mine. *What is her name?* I tell her the whole story without remembering her name, and she hugs me fiercely and says she's so glad I'm doing better, and then she looks me in the eye and asks, "Can I tell, like, everyone in the neighborhood about this?" and I say sure, because that will save me from explaining, if I ever run into anyone, and they'll all know what happened without having to ask me "What happened?" while I stand there pausing and saying "Well . . ." as I try to gauge what's easiest to say.

She says goodbye, and I continue on my way, but after standing and talking for so long, I'm exhausted. My brain tires so easily of telling stories, of understanding stories. It needs so much rest, and stories demand so much energy.

I don't mean to be an unreliable narrator, but sometimes that's what happens.

Sometimes I say, "I had a tough year, but it's better now."

Sometimes I say, "Oh, the kids, they're doing great. What about yours?"

Sometimes I say, "Yeah, I had a weird thing happen with my brain, but it's okay now, I think it's fixed, it could be fixed, or I might have to go back, I don't know yet, I just kind of have to wait and see, I'll only know if I'm better if I stop being better, if it stops working, if I start leaking again, if the headache returns, then I'll be able to say, oh, I was better for a while, but otherwise I just have to wait and hope my headache stays in the front of my head and not in back, and that I don't get another cold and cough or sneeze, or bend over too far, or twist, or lift something that's a little too heavy, but at least this time if it gets bad again, if I start leaking again, I know where to go, and I can just talk to the doctors there and go back again to get fixed."

Sometimes I say, "Good, I'm good. How are you?"

Rebound intracranial hypertension (RIH) is a potential complication of epidural blood patching characterized by a postprocedural elevation of CSF pressure . . . . The mechanism underlying this phenomenon remains unknown and the onset of symptoms has been reported over a wide timeframe, ranging from days to years after [epidural blood patch]. Despite the small number of reported cases in the literature, our experience has been that this phenomenon is not uncommon. It is likely, in our opinion, that RIH often goes unrecognized.

The primary clinical manifestation of RIH is headache, which may be accompanied by nausea, emesis, and blurred vision. Because patients with [spontaneous intracranial hypotension] typically also have headache as their primary complaint, and because experience with treating these patients is limited at many centers, the headaches associated with RIH might be mistakenly attributed to refractory [spontaneous intracranial hypotension]. As a consequence, treatment aimed at increasing CSF pressure, such as repeat [epidural blood patches], will be unhelpful for patients with RIH and could even exacerbate the condition. Awareness of this complication is therefore important.

—P.G. Kranz, T.J. Amrhein, and L. Gray, "Rebound Intracranial Hypertension: A Complication of Epidural Blood Patching for Intracranial Hypotension," *American Journal of Neuroradiology, June 2014*

30

February 2016

R ebound, like *spontaneous*, is a funny word. There is an energy
to it, a buoyancy, a lightness that seems to imply a temporary
state, the moment just after you spring off a trampoline and hover,
nearly weightless, in the air, and just before you land again, sinking
down into the elastic place that launches you ever upwards. *Rebound*
makes me think of relationships, the fling you have to get over
the guy who broke your heart, and in that sense it carries with it a
feeling of propulsion, of abandon, an almost predatory or at least
pointed and specific kind of freedom. It makes me think of flying,
after having been on the ground. Potential energy suddenly made
potent.

But my rebound high pressure is neither high-flying nor short-lived. It is a constant thing, my leap from the depths of those leaking days a launch into slow-motion suspension, a tense floating that seems to defy gravity as I pause mid-flight, high, my head tight with fluid.

Imagine you are on an airplane, and imagine that you have a cold, or a sinus infection, and imagine that during the plane's descent the pilot is required to circle for a bit before landing, and imagine that that altitude where the plane kills time is precisely the level of altitude that makes your sinus pressure unbearable. Your face hurts, your head hurts, it feels as though the front of your face is encased in pain. Perhaps you feel nauseated from it, perhaps the other passengers notice you crying. You can't pop your ears to release the pressure, in fact there is no release, until finally, thankfully, the pilot announces the plane has been cleared to make its final descent, and moves down, down, closer to the ground, away from the altitude level that held your head in a vise.

That's what rebound high pressure is like, here on the ground, at sea level, in my house, in my room, in my bed. Caffeine makes it worse, salt makes it worse, sitting makes it worse, lying flat makes it worse. Afternoons make it worse, because that's when cerebrospinal fluid production bottoms out, and the middle of the night makes it worse, because that's when cerebrospinal fluid production surges again. My choroid plexus has been producing cerebrospinal fluid, circulating it and swelling it and creating a high tide in the dead of night and a low tide in the late afternoon, since before I even had a brain. And yet until now I've never noticed, never been sensitive to the high tides of the ocean in my head.

When it's bad, when I forget and have caffeine or a salty food, or lie down in my bed without the wedge pillow to prop me up, or even when I've done nothing to provoke it except be alive with a brain now sensitive to the ebb and flow of fluid, I feel not only the tightness in my head, the headache in the front of my head, behind my eyes, on the top of my forehead, I feel a heaviness and burning along my spine, just between my shoulder blades, where it's theorized the leak likely was. I lean on ice packs, long and cold against my spine. Will this surge pry open the wound? Will the rising tide of fluid seep into the edges of the patched-up tear, like the rain that finds its way into my house sometimes, trickling through the brick, inexorably flowing toward a weak, leaky spot?

Little is understood about rebound intracranial hypertension, even by neurologists and other doctors who work with headache patients. It's generally noted as a new headache that develops after blood patching—which is confusing, since most people who receive blood patches are being treated for headaches in the first place. The rebound headache often has a different quality than the leak headache, though—frontal instead of occipital, worse instead of better when lying down, sometimes accompanied by nausea and vomiting and blurry vision—and while it generally develops within hours or days after patching, sometimes it can be weeks or even months until the headache reveals itself. The severity of these rebound headaches is not dependent on the volume of blood in the blood patch a patient receives; a patient can experience painful rebound intracranial hypertension regardless of whether they've been injected with 5 ccs of blood or 30. And there are some patients who receive large-volume blood patches and don't experience rebound high pressure at all.

It is all very much still a mystery why this happens to some patients and not others, why for some patients this is a state that persists for months or even years after successful patching. Even physiological explanations are merely theories at this point. One thought is that perhaps the blood injected to the epidural space during a blood patch acts like a kind of blood pressure cuff, squeezing the thecal sac (also called the dural sac, the protective membrane sur-rounding the spinal cord) and displacing the cerebrospinal fluid within it upward from the spinal canal and into the head. And yet this doesn't explain the rebound symptoms of the patient who's given 5 ccs of blood—which is not enough to squeeze or compress anything, really—or the complete lack of rebound symptoms in a patient who's given 30 ccs—which is more than enough to produce pressure on the thecal sac.

Another thought is that compensatory cerebrospinal fluid production—the body's overproduction of CSF to compensate for a leak—may be a factor. While the volume of blood used in blood patching is not a predictor of who may or may not develop rebound high pressure, one factor might be: the length of time a patient has been dealing with a spinal CSF leak. While a person is leaking, their body's natural CSF production is increased to compensate for the leak, and the longer a person has been leaking and thus overcompensating, the longer it may take for the brain and body to adjust to more normal levels once the leak is patched. This is the hose and faucet metaphor I used to explain to my children about my new headache situation after I returned home from the pro-cedure they'd expected to cure me of my constant headache, and it makes a lot of intuitive sense. But that doesn't fully explain the phenomenon either.

Another thought is that people's anatomy varies, and some people's dura and veins are more compliant, more resilient, than others. Physiological things happen in people with spinal CSF leaks, and one of those things is that while leaking, the epidural venous plexus (a network of veins that extends from the skull base to the sacrum) dilates, meaning all those veins expand and become engorged, to compensate for the lower levels of cerebrospinal fluid. The elasticity and capacity for dilation in epidural and cranial veins varies from person to person, and that may explain why some people suffer more from rebound high pressure than others—some people's veins may be able to dilate more without triggering any pain. The dura, too, varies: Although its medical name translates to "tough mother," the toughness of it isn't always uniform throughout in one person's body, and the toughness or flexibility of one person's dura can be different from the toughness or flexibility of another's. Along these same lines, one person's baseline CSF pressure may be much lower than another person's, and so what's high for the first person is normal-feeling for the second. Dr. Kranz explained this to me using the metaphor of a balloon: "It could be that you have a pressure of ten, and I boost it to eighteen, and then you have symptoms of rebound intracranial hypertension. But then here comes somebody off the street and I measure their pressure and they're eighteen. You both have a pressure of eighteen, and yet you're symptomatic and they're not. Why is that? It may have something to do with the elasticity of the system. The person off the street, whose pressure is eighteen, may have a dura like a latex balloon that can expand and contract—but if your pressure is eighteen and your dura is like a Mylar balloon, we've pushed you to your limit. So every time you cough or bend over, or turn your head the wrong way or sit for too long, you're pushing against a rigid system."

In a small study Dr. Kranz and his team did at Duke, they found that of thirty patients with spinal CSF leaks who received blood or fibrin glue patches, about a third of those patients had no rebound intracranial hypotension symptoms afterward, 43 percent had mild symptoms (treated with Tylenol and head elevation), 17 percent had moderate symptoms (treated with Diamox, usually administered orally, though in some cases via IV), and two patients had symptoms severe enough that they had to go back to the hospital and have their spinal fluid drained to get back to normal levels. These were all patients who were followed and treated based on their symptoms within days of their patches, and even with that kind of close monitoring, treating rebound high pressure is tricky, and varies from patient to patient. For doctors without much experience in treating post-patching rebound headaches in patients with CSF leaks, especially those patients whose rebound headaches develop months afterward instead of days afterward, it can be a real challenge.

In the beginning, in the early weeks post-patching, this rebound pressure is a constant state for me, one that makes me long for the days of the leak, when lying down brought some relief, at least, however minimal, however short-lived. The rebound headache, when it surges, can't be soothed the same way. The only thing that brings relief is time, waiting it out, surviving it. I also don't fully understand it, I don't understand why I still have this constant pain; although I've come up with that hose analogy to explain it somewhat to my kids, I haven't fully absorbed the meaning of it for myself, I haven't yet read about the mechanisms of rebound high pressure, I haven't yet thought through what it is that these pain signals are trying to communicate, I haven't learned yet by going where I need to go.

And so, when I check in with my neurologist at the headache center about a month after my patch procedure, and she suggests coming back in for another round of infusion treatment to help ease the pain of this new constant post-leak-patching headache, I don't think about how the word *infusion* means *the pouring in of liquid*, about how the process involves introducing bag after bag of saline and liquid medicine into my veins. I don't think about how right now this pain is happening because my veins are already full, engorged and stretched to their limit, how it's happening because everything is at full capacity. Instead I think, *pain relief*, and so I say yes, and I schedule the appointment. I return to the infusion center, I sign all the papers, I approve all the medications, I climb into the comfortable recliner and have prewarmed blankets laid over me, I am hooked up to the IV.

Within minutes of starting, I feel worse. My head feels swollen, packed with cotton, stuffed to the breaking point, and I am nauseated, eye-blurred, forehead-stabbed. I adjust the recliner so that I'm tilted at an angle, my head elevated, but the pain gets worse. I call the nurse in and tell her I'm feeling bad, that whatever they're giving me is making me feel terrible. She looks confused and somewhat dubious as she tells me that so far all I've gotten is saline. *Saline.* A part of me makes the connection, a part of me thinks *Hello, that is salt and water, and isn't salt the enemy right now, doesn't salt make everything terrible, doesn't salt give you a headache now and make your head try to explode?* But then the Benadryl and lorazepam start to kick in and I become very sleepy, and I tell the nurse, "I don't think I can do this, this isn't helping," but I'm also drifting off, and I hear her tell me that we can check in after this round of treatment, that we can reevaluate at lunchtime, and if I still feel awful, we can stop.

By lunchtime, even with all the pain-fighting medicine coursing through my veins, I am miserable. My high-pressure headache is higher and more pressurized than it has been since the day after I was first patched, and I am beginning to realize what a mistake this was for me to do this. Why did my neurologist think this would help? Why did I? I sign myself out of the infusion center at lunchtime, woozy with pain and pain medicine, and cancel the next day's appointment, the second part of the two-day process. Once home, I post to the rebound high-pressure leaker group, text with my leaker friends, "Oh yeah," they all agree, "you're in rebound high pressure right now! That kind of infusion thing will only make your rebound headache worse! Saline! Pumping fluids into you when you're already sensitive to changes in fluid pressure!" If only I'd consulted them before I'd decided to do this. If only my neurologist had understood this. "Take an over-the-counter diuretic," they advise me. "Drink dandelion tea." "If you have to lie down, use the wedge pillow and keep your head elevated at thirty degrees." "Use an ice pack."

I do these things. I drink dandelion tea, I wear my ice turban; I stand, since sitting or lying down makes it worse, even though standing is still exhausting; I use my wedge pillow when I lie down. I quibble with the insurance company, which has billed me for both days, even though I left after half of one. It takes weeks for this infusion, this surge, to resolve, for my body to calm itself. I have rebounded, and this time the bounding part of it happens in slow motion, suspending me in midair, at the altitude of pain.

Gradually, the rebound gains a rhythm to it, begins to have its own ebb and flow over time. The infusion-induced spike fades back to the levels of my post-patching rebound high, and gradually my rebound high-pressure peaks become monthly, tied to my cycle, rather than daily—a week or so of terrible face headache and pressure fading back into the new normal of low-level face headache and pressure.

It's comforting, in its own way, as nerve-racking as it is to have this constant anxiety of wondering if today will be the day that the pressure will be too much, will rip through the fragile reconstitution of my dura, will tear through the torn place. It's comforting because, as worrisome as it is, as long as I have the high-pressure headache, I know that I'm not leaking. The rebound high pressure is proof that it's working, that the seal is holding, that the leak is patched, however tenuous the patching may be.

Eventually, over time, this rebound high pressure will dissipate, the daily peaks becoming monthly peaks, becoming every-few-months peaks, becoming peaks that exist only when I forget and sit too long, or have too many Diet Cokes, or eat a too-salty thing.

Eventually, this rebound will align itself more with its proper definition, which is: to bounce back.

31

When you first begin piano lessons, time is a strict thing. The metronome is a looming wooden triangle on the music rack, a strange-looking clock, its one thin arm marking time by swinging faster or slower depending on where the adjustable weight is slid on the pendulum, a satisfying yet ominous, demanding, mechanical click emanating from it as it sets the tempo. Or it is a small rectangular plastic box leaning against the score before you, a dial to set the speed, a blinking light and digital click sound to alert you to the tempo. Or, now, it is an app on a phone, purely digital, a simulacrum of the old clockwork device, a visual thing, a movie of a metronome, a screen you slide and tap to set the pace, the volume. Whatever form it takes, the keeping and marking of time is exact and unforgiving, and a mainstay of early piano training. Scales and arpeggios become governed by the metronome's unrelenting precision. Tricky passages of repertoire are practiced at slow metronomic speeds, the weight or dial or slider gradually moved to increase tempo as the passage at slower speeds is mastered. All of this to help the pianist internalize a sense of time, to help bring awareness to the places where there is a tendency to slow down, to race ahead. All of this to help regulate.

In the beginning, this is to help establish what time feels like, to bring awareness to the differences between the experience of internal time and the reality of external time, the differences between what you hear in your head while sitting at the instrument and what listeners hear while sitting across the room from you when you play. And for that purpose, time is strict, mathematical, precise. Deviation from tempo is a mistake to be corrected, whether it's slowing down because a passage is too tricky for a beginner's fingers to manage at full speed, or speeding up because of the excitement of momentum, your fingers a perpetual motion machine becoming increasingly faster and in danger of crashing to a halt. Being grounded in time helps you bridge the gap between what you feel when you play and what people hear when you play it. It helps the player become a reliable narrator, a performer in control of the material, putting an audience at ease through the regularity of tempo, no inconsistent slowing and surging, no speeding up like a runaway train.

But later you learn—after years of having precision and stability and predictability and consistency ingrained in your fingers, your muscles, your ears, your brain, your body—that time is not strict, or rather that there is fluidity within its structure. It's a bit like the moment you discover, after thinking for so long that numbers are static and progressive and inviolable, that one comes after zero and two comes after one, and that's the way it works, that there is actually an infinity of numbers between zero and one, and one and two, and so on. There is an infinity of time between notes, no matter how rigidly the metronome insists otherwise, beating on and on, exactly so, and the job of a true musician is to understand how to play with that time, how to manipulate that time, how to play within it.

There is a law of conservation with time and music, just as there is with physics. The total time of a piece remains constant, and yet the time within it—stretching out a phrase for emphasis, condensing a passage to heighten its impact—is fluid. Any time you take from one place—slowing nearly imperceptibly as you resolve a chord, for instance—must be made up in another, otherwise the performance would be as rambling and uncontrolled and ramshackled and unpracticed as a beginner's who doesn't understand the importance of the larger consistency of time, and who thus cannot respect the infinities within it. But to be able to take those liberties, you must have a solid basis, a solid grounding, not only in the practical, literal, written score, but in the body, in the practiced muscles and ears and brain.

Early practice, the first approaches to a piece of music, if it's done smartly and with an eye toward building a performance from a solid foundation, takes into account this fluidity of time, this infinity between each note, because early practice is slow practice. If revision is the heart of writing, then slow practice is the heart of playing. In slow practice, you can savor time, because you are outside of time. You can sink into each note, each chord, and allow your muscles to relax into place, allow your brain to align its pathways, new connections forming as you repeat and replay, because this, too, is the hallmark of early practice, and of being outside of time. Repetition, and slowness, and the gradual learning and relearning and telling and retelling of a pattern, of a process, of a progression.

This kind of work, this slow, deliberate work, outside of time but decidedly within it, taking place over a passage of time, is like recovery.

It is a kind of healing.

I have been outside of time, even as time passes, for so long with this illness, and with this recovery. Time, when I was leaking, was stasis: the ceiling above my bed, the walls of my room, nothing changing as I lay flat day after day. And yet all around me time was passing. I could hear the low whoosh of cars driving past outside my windows, the clock tower bells from City Hall chiming toward me some quiet days. My children, growing taller, becoming more and more themselves every day, outgrowing their clothes, their faces acquiring cheekbones, morphing into adult shapes. Nothing stopped merely because I stopped being able to participate in it. Even within my own body time continued its pace, blood circulating, fingernails growing, hair graying, monthly cycle cycling, all the cycles cycling of sleeping and waking and hunger and elimination. So I was suspended in time even as time continued around me and within me, I floated in the infinity between one note and the next, between one number and the next.

Can a self exist outside of time? When I was leaking, I felt as if I had no self. Or rather that the self I thought I always had been, and that had always been in charge, was in fact revealed to be a fiction, as imaginary and theoretical as in-between-numbers infinity. I had made the rookie mistake of confusing my mind for my brain: I thought that "I" was the driver of all my thoughts and decisions and actions. But, deprived of enough cerebrospinal fluid for my mind to function properly though my brain continued its work, it became clear that this "I," this self, this mind, was no driver at all, that in fact the proper mechanical analogy might be that if my body is a car, my brain is the driver, and my mind, in fact, is merely a passenger. This makes me think of two things: of the amusement park rides where you "drive" cars, which in fact are entirely programmed to go where they need to go, without your doing anything at all; and of a toddler, sitting in a car seat, in the back of the car, with a pretend steering wheel, imagining that he is driving the big machine. My self, my mind, all along, has been this deluded passenger, this backseat driver, while my brain and body oblige it, allowing it to believe it's in charge while they continue their work.

Stuck in time, my mind is exposed as a thing entirely separate from the ongoing duties of my brain. Recovering means integrating these things, rejoining time. Returning to the myth of myself as the true driver.

In real life, I don't drive at all. I walk everywhere. If I need to go someplace far, I use an app to summon a car service.

I don't even have a driver's license.

Rests do not mean "to rest," my piano teacher told me, back when I was still a teenager, at the conservatory, learning how to think about music, about art. *This an opportunity to stop time, prepare. Sometimes savor. Do you know what this means, stop time? You hurry, hurry. But there is time. Feel it. Rest means active. There is music even in the waiting, even in the silence.*

I still hurry, hurry. I still resist rest, I still resist stopping time. But right now resting is required, mandatory. Not just by doctor's orders, but by my brain. I sleep so much, I need so much sleep. Being awake is exhausting, talking and thinking is exhausting. Reading a paragraph or two requires a nap. But I think about what she said, about this being an opportunity to prepare, in the stopped time; about the way resting can be active; about how there is music in the waiting, in the silence. And I try to be patient with it instead of fight it. I try to savor.

I am in the slow-practice phase, I realize, in my life. Repetition and slowness. The learning and relearning of what I am capable of as I heal. The telling and retelling myself and others of this story, to make sense of what has happened and what continues to happen and what might happen. The gradual process of a progression toward baseline, which is both a return to a place and an entirely new destination.

Eventually I will play with time again, stretch it out and compress it, find the places to lightly rush and to deliberately languish. For now I am in the process of sinking into the slow, measured phrase, learning to allow my brain to think in time again, each day a slow tick of the metronome as I reengage with the practice of living.

Pain, as a submodality of somatic sensation, has been defined as a "complex constellation of unpleasant sensory, emotional and cognitive experiences provoked by real or perceived tissue damage and manifested by certain autonomic, psychological, and behavioral reactions." . . . Pain is described as having different qualities and temporal features depending on the modality and locality of the stimulus, respectively: first pain is described as lancinating, stabbing, or pricking; second pain is more pervasive and includes burning, throbbing, cramping, and aching and recruits sustained affective components with descriptors such as "sickening." The intensity of these global reactions underscores the importance of avoiding damaging situations for survival and maintaining homeostasis. As opposed to the relatively more objective nature of other senses, pain is highly individual and subjective, and the translation of nociception into pain perception can be curtailed by stress or exacerbated by anticipation.

—Adrienne E. Dubin and Ardem Patapoutian,
"Nociceptors: The Sensors of the Pain Pathway,"
The Journal of Clinical Investigation, November 2010

32

March 2016

B ack at the headache center for a follow-up visit, I fill out the
same old questionnaire: *Are there any events that have affected
your headache? Have you had any headache-free periods? On a scale of
0–10, how severe are your headaches? Have your headache symptoms or
location changed?*

There are no questions that are tailored to my own particular
experience of having a spinal CSF leak and getting it patched,
no inquiries about pain that take into account my particular circumstance. Each time I must explain to the doctors I see that
the headaches I have now and the kinds of pain I'm experiencing
exist as a reaction to the procedure I had done and the amount of

intracranial pressure I'm sensing now that my cerebrospinal fluid isn't leaking out anymore.

Headache pain of any kind, especially headache pain that is chronic, is still a mystery for doctors and patients alike. "Headache" is a description of what's happening, rather than a description of what's going wrong in the body. And *pain*, from the Greek *poine*, meaning "penalty," from the Latin *poena*, which means "punishment"; pain itself is of course subjective. Pain feels like a penalty, like a punishment, the price you pay for a message from your body that something's not right. Sometimes this punishment can be deferred, as in those times of immense adrenaline-rushing stress, when you don't notice the pain of an injury until after the intensity and immediacy of the moment has passed; and sometimes this punishment builds upon itself so much that, rather than your being able to delay the sensation of it, you become overly sensitive to it, and it no longer takes the same amount of pain for you to experience the sensation of pain at all. Pain becomes its own cycle of sensation, almost separate from the original bodily signals that provoked it in the first place.

Throughout the process of my dura leaking cerebrospinal fluid, my main, most durable, notable symptom was pain: omnipresent, chronic, and overwhelming, and located, seemingly, in my head. And yet my CSF leak was not itself located in my head. I didn't have a cranial leak, but my pain was entirely within my cranium, almost exclusively focused in the right side of the back of my skull. Part of why the pain of headaches is particularly confounding is because while the experience of pain usually has a localized nature, or at least feels like it exists in a certain spot, like my CSF leak headache, exactly where those pain signals originate from is not straightforward. Pain sensation in the head is generally transmitted via nerves that all bundle together in the region of the spinal trigeminal nucleus, a cluster of neurons that receive information about touch, pain, and temperature from cranial nerves including the trigeminal nerve, the facial nerve, the glossopharyngeal nerve, and the vagus nerve. This tangled bundle of nerves is part of why the precise cause of headaches can be difficult to isolate, and why pain felt in certain parts of the head can in fact be generated from locations elsewhere in the head and body.

There are a few theories about what exactly causes headache pain in people with spinal CSF leaks. The most obvious one is the loss of cerebrospinal fluid and the resulting lowered intracranial pressure: When a person with a spinal CSF leak stands up, that loss of brain buoyancy, and the effects of gravity while a person is upright and the brain shifts downward, can put pressure on pain-sensitive structures in the head and neck. Another theory is based on what's called the Monro-Kellie hypothesis (named for the two eighteenth-century Scottish physicians who coined it), which posits that within the rigid compartment of the skull, there is a constant pressure-volume relationship between the brain, cerebrospinal fluid, and intracranial blood. A decrease in any one of those three things is compensated by an increase in the others. When the amount of cerebrospinal fluid is lower than normal, due to a leak, this volume has to be made up somehow. Brain tissue can't really expand, at least as far as we know; and so what happens is the intracranial blood vessels start to dilate, to compensate for the lack of cerebrospinal fluid. This expansion of arteries and veins, which increases rapidly when a leaking person stands up, can be a painful sensation.

Another explanation of what causes pain in people with spinal CSF leaks involves the notion of compliance, or craniospinal elasticity. Just as some individual people can be more psychologically resilient than others, individual people's physical anatomies can be more resilient than others (such as in Dr. Kranz's example of the dural sacs of two different hypothetical people with the same level of spinal fluid pressure, one of whom has a dura that is flexible like a latex balloon, and one whose dura is more rigid, like a Mylar balloon). The headache pain that is such a hallmark of spinal cerebrospinal fluid leaks may come from changes in compliance. The amount of compliance or flexibility within the cranial space is limited, since it's a closed space covered by an unyielding, impenetrable skull: The intracranial blood vessels can dilate, as in the Monro-Kellie hypothesis, but there's only so much room for expansion. In the lumbar region, however, there's more room to expand, as there's no skull to contain it, only the self-limiting capacity of the tough (but more flexible than bone) dura. So there is a contradiction: the dura tight and noncompliant in the cranial space, with veins dilating and becoming stiffer, more engorged with fluid; and the dura looser and more floppy in the lumbar space, where there's more room to expand, and where, due to gravity and a leak preventing the normal flow and circulation of spinal fluid, the fluid can collect, stretching and straining the dura mater. This contradiction, this interruption of the normally uniform distribution of craniospinal elasticity, can be a factor in causing headache pain.

The dura mater in general is not a stretchy thing, and although it accommodates changes in fluid pressure, it's not elastic in the way we think of a rubber band or a bouncy ball being elastic. While I was leaking, the dura was explained to me in many different ways. I heard it described as a thin covering, like a cloth. I heard it described as a hollow plastic tube. I was told it was like packing tape, the kind with strings throughout it for added toughness and durability. I was told it was like duct tape, the super strong and sticky kind that's hard to puncture. I was told it was a kind of connective tissue, which it is, and not a muscle, which it is not, and that it wasn't something I could either strengthen or diminish through exercise or physical therapy. But what I didn't realize was that this tube, as thin as cloth, as tough as packing tape, is, as yet another doctor explained, richly endowed with nociceptive fibers. Which means that this plastic tube encasing the brain and spinal cord is capable of sensing and transmitting pain.

Nociceptive is a word that comes from the Latin *nocere*, "to harm," and what it describes is a kind of receptor in a sensory neuron that detects and responds to unpleasant stimuli in the body by sending electrical signals to the central nervous system. We have these kinds of nociceptors all over our bodies, and the electrical signals they send to the spinal cord and brain alert us to possible threats, and to harmful sensations. Think of your fingers touching a hot surface: In an instant, the nociceptive fibers in your skin send the message to your brain that there is danger, and before you can even form the thought, *Ouch, this is hot,* your hand has already jerked away to safety from that hot place. Those particular fast-acting fibers (called A-delta nociceptor fibers) are large in diameter and have a thick myelin sheath surrounding them, which enables them to conduct nerve impulses more speedily than other fibers. They are the messengers texting your brain with the immediacy of the event, a live Twitter feed of pain. Now think of your fingers after having touched the hot surface: They're away and out of danger, and the sharp, quick, specific pain of that initial contact is gone; but now you are left with the duller, throbbing, more diffuse and longer-lasting pain of the place where your skin is slightly burned. This kind of pain is brought to you by slower-acting fibers, called C fibers, which are much smaller in diameter and take much longer to communicate messages—rather than Tweeting at your brain with urgency, they are writing a letter and mailing it. These slower, more deliberate C fibers account for about 70 percent of all nociceptive fibers. And the dull, aching pain of headache, as seen in headache disorders—from cluster headaches to spinal CSF leaks—seems to be communicated by these fibers.

The dura, with its nociceptive fibers, is sensitive to traction, and traction can translate into pain. When I was leaking, when I experienced a headache upon standing, theoretically part of the reason for this was the decrease in my already low intracranial cerebrospinal fluid volume due to the new gravity of being upright, plus the stretching or traction of the dura as it responded to the contents of my skull shifting downward, however slightly. As I'm recovering from this leak, my dura is still hypersensitive, all its nociceptors on high alert, ever at the ready, waiting for the smallest of signals, and so my pain now is from the volume of cerebrospinal fluid reaching full capacity, from the traction on the dura caused by tilting my chin, from the way it is stretched simply by my sitting down. All of this stimuli, which previously, in my non-leaking life, was merely interpreted by my body as stimuli—not danger, not threat, not pain—is now transmitted as signals of peril. My brain is sensitized, my pain pathways are sensitized, and so the pain cycle continues.

Sensitization is an important component of pain. It is an increased response to stimuli, which results in both increased sensitivity to pain and the experience of previously non-painful things now being experienced as painful. As I recover from my leak, with my sensitized dura, I am painfully sensitive to the pulsation and circulation of spinal fluid as I never have been before, despite the fact that my spinal fluid has been pulsating and circulating my whole life. And while I was leaking, I became sensitized to that pain as well: After a while it took longer and longer for the pain brought on by being upright to subside once I lay flat. My pain was continuous, even in the absence of painful input. This kind of sensitization is in part why techniques like the infusion treatments I had at the headache center are prescribed: Those several days of concentrated exposure to medications, some to constrict blood vessels, some to induce relaxation, all to decrease pain, help to interrupt the pain cycle, to reset things so that these sensitive receptors can recalibrate, and return to their normal levels of sensitivity.

The main difference between the pain I had while leaking and the pain I have now is that the pain I have now changes over time. It is intermittent, and variable in intensity. I can answer the headache center questionnaire questions like *Have you had any headache-free periods?* because now that answer, incredibly, is *yes*. I can quantify the number of headache hours I have each day, because now my headache is not continuous, it is not intractable; it has a cycle to it that is no longer dependent upon whether or not I am standing. The questions of scale that confounded me with my leak headache—*On a scale of 0-10, how severe are your headaches? __/10 Mild ones __/10 Severe ones __/10 Average ones*—are fathomable now that my headache (singular, unceasing) has become headaches (plural, limited in duration), now that I have moments when my head hurts less than it does in other moments. This is progress, and I note it, tracking each day on an app on my phone, so that eventually I can see that what feels like stasis is in fact an evolution, my pain waxing and waning, ebbing and flowing, my fast and slow nerve fibers recalibrating themselves, until eventually, one day, it might even be gone.

33

It's happened again: I've forgotten something crucial—the pro-phylactic medication, an antidote, a cure—and now we are all at risk. I sit up in bed, but it's already too late. I can see the laser beams cutting through the ceiling, brilliant sparks penetrating the darkness, and then the poison gas begins seeping in through the floor. Soon the house will shake and collapse upon us. It's only a matter of time. My throat burns. I clutch at my neck, gagging, choking, as I search fruitlessly on the dresser, the nightstand, for the thing that surely must be there to protect me, the mask or the pill or the whatever it was I was supposed to have prepared in order to save us. But it's not there, of course it's not there, nothing's there, I've failed as I always fail, as I'm destined to do every time, and so I run to the hallway, screaming as I throw open my bedroom door, the panic propelling me, my heart a rapid staccato in my throat. *I've got to get the kids before it's too late, I've got to save them, I've got to get them out.*

Suddenly, standing in the harsh light of the hallway, I feel myself beginning to wake up, the pain in the back of my head dawning, and the truth slowly returns to me: There is no disaster. There are no deadly lasers cutting through my roof and destroying my house, no deadly gas flowing through the vents. This is a nightmare. A night terror.

I'm not in danger; I'm standing halfway down the stairs in the middle of the night, the cats circling my feet, confused and yet hopeful that it might already be food time, my son sleepily calling from his room, "You okay?" I'm shaking, my breath ragged with adrenaline, my mind still half-convinced the terror was real, that it really might be real, while another part of me knows it couldn't be. "Sorry," I say. "Nightmare." I take a few more breaths and return to my bedroom. The lights are on somehow, I must have slapped the wall switch in my panicked run out of the room, and I sink down onto the bed, still shaky, still confused, and finally see the note I left for myself next to my bed before I fell asleep, a message in all caps, written in ballpoint pen thickened to readable status by retracing many times the outline of the letters: "IT'S. NOT. REAL."

I see it, I read it, I recognize it as a letter from my waking self to my panicked dreaming self; and yet it seems possible that it's wrong. Perhaps this is still part of the nightmare. I sit holding the note, reading those three words, trying to convince myself that they're true, that it was a dream, that none of it was real, until finally it feels believable enough to turn off the lights and lie down again. My pulse races, even while I lie still and try to calm my breathing, but eventually I'm able to fall asleep.

∽

Leaving myself a note was one of the many things I tried in my attempts to thwart the night terrors. I wrote one that said: "Remember, this is only a dream." I wrote another that said: "You're dreaming." And of course there was the frantic but direct "IT'S. NOT. REAL." I placed these in various spots near my bed before going to sleep, in the hope that reading them in the midst of a nightmare would help me cut through the panic and bewilderment; but usually I would discover them only after fully waking, the screaming and running and occasionally ankle-twisting midnight anxiety attack already over.

I tried reciting calming affirmations before going to sleep for the night, lying still and doing the kind of breathing I'd learned years before in ashtanga yoga class, each inhalation and exhalation an audible, strong force in my throat. *Everything is fine*, I'd tell myself. *You'll go to sleep and sleep all night, you'll wake up in the morning after a peaceful rest.* I tried listening to soothing binaural soundtracks, supposedly calibrated to send your brain into relaxed states through sounds that triggered delta waves, gamma waves, electrical currents designed to induce tranquility. Still, despite my preparations, I would find myself again fending off the inevitable attack, waking up my children, startling the cats, scaring myself as I'd wake up in the process of running out of my room, down the stairs, trying to escape.

These nighttime episodes are terrifying as they happen, but in retrospect almost embarrassingly obvious. There's no clever symbolism to my nightmares, no mystery to solve or truth to decode, just the panic and terror of having forgotten something crucial. It's the panic of things left undone, the terror that my own forgetful, foggy brain has doomed us. The creeping worry that I have damaged my children beyond repair with my divorcing their father, with my malfunctioning brain, with my inability to do the things I have always done for them.

"Have you experienced this sort of thing before?" my neurologist asked when I'd finally told her about the night terrors, seven months into my CSF leak, before getting patched up at Duke. "Not like this," I'd said. It's true that years before, when I'd been on a punishing deadline with a difficult co-worker, I'd had stressful dreams, nightmares about the walls literally closing in—but this is how all my dreams are, even the non-scary ones: overly obvious, no interpretive skills necessary, no insight required. "Huh," she'd said. "Maybe it could be stress? Are you stressed about something?" For a moment, I'd thought she was joking. "I mean . . ." I'd begun, gesturing at myself, sitting in a neurologist's office in a headache center at a brain hospital, slumped down in a chair not made for slumping, in an attempt to be as flat as I could possibly be to mitigate the effects of my own brain fluid leaking out of my head. *Yes???*

Emi had night terrors when she was three, a moment in time after Nate was born, but before she was able to connect the dots between that event and the stress she felt because of it. Night terrors are common in children, according to the parenting books I read at the time, especially in toddlers. The advice for parents is to stay calm and not try to wake them; to put yourself between them and anything dangerous, but to not attempt to restrain them or hold them, as this may agitate them more. It was unsettling and distressing to have to merely watch her suffer through these episodes, trying to soothe her and reassure her without physically interfering, unable to snap her out of her panic and back to reality. Often, even though her eyes would be open, she would in fact be asleep the whole time. She never had any memory of these nightmares upon waking.

I did, though; her cries haunted me. Every time she had one of these night terrors, it was the same anguish: She was calling out for her mommy, panicked that she couldn't find her mommy, that she had lost her mommy. And yet when I would go to her, telling her "Shh, shh, it's Mommy, I'm here, I'm right here, you didn't lose me, I'm right here with you," that would make it worse. Her eyes—wide open, but unseeing—would flash with panic and she would scream, "You're not my mommy, I need my *real* mommy." In the daytime, I would understand this as her way of processing the grief of losing her mommy to this new interloper of a baby brother, her instinctive sadness and fear that our relationship would change. Her "real" mommy was a mommy only to her, her and her alone, and that's what she was desperately searching for in the middle of the night, that's the loss she was grieving: the loss of having me all to herself. But in the dark, in the middle of the night, in her room, trying to comfort her, I worried maybe she was onto something. Perhaps she had seen right through me, perhaps her wild eyes had seen the truth: I wasn't a real mother, I was a faker; I was ambivalent, and my ambivalence was causing me to fail her.

Her night terrors subsided after several months, as the parenting books said they would, and did not return. She had the occasional nightmare from time to time, but nothing like the awake-but-asleep episodes she'd had while adjusting to Nate's existence, and the question of whether or not I was a real enough mother for her was put to rest, for the time being.

Unlike Emi, I remembered my night-terror episodes in my waking hours, and they struck me as being a comically exaggerated shadow version of a process that unfolded in my daily life, as I lay in bed, trying to retrace my steps and find my way back to the moment that started it all. Just like in the nightmares, which were only slight variations on the same theme every night, I kept finding myself endlessly revisiting the series of events that had resulted in my ending up where I was. *If I hadn't gotten sick. If I hadn't left the house. If I hadn't coughed.* No matter how many ways I tried to think about it, I was inevitably led to the same conclusion, which was that it didn't matter how I thought about it or how I understood it: It had happened. Knowing exactly how or why wouldn't help me, wouldn't heal the tear in my dura, wouldn't stop the leak or prevent the pain or undo the damage done. And yet I'd find myself returning there in my thoughts, such as they were, the same way I'd find myself awake in the night, on the landing or the stairs or in my bathroom, my chest tight with fear, battling against the inevitable nocturnal disaster.

I continued my pre-bedtime self-talk. I took the advice of my sister Jessie, who recommended setting an alarm to wake myself just before I slipped into the sleep phase that somehow sparked the nightmare scenarios for me, usually within a few hours of my falling asleep for the night. I wrote more notes to myself, I listened to calming music and guided meditation, I fell asleep to peaceful, tranquil sounds. I tried, variously and with little success, Benadryl, trazodone, melatonin, lorazepam, alcohol.

I listened to a podcast one night where a man shared his story of surviving a terrible accident and how he coped with the night terrors that were part of his PTSD. He said that instead of replaying the story of the accident for himself, he began to try to rewrite it. Before going to sleep, he'd talk himself through what happened—except instead of the tragic ending, he would turn the events of the day that changed his life into just a regular, boring, ordinary day. He still woke up confronting the reality of being partially paralyzed—that would never change; but the night terrors stopped holding him in their grip.

This made sense to me, this idea of changing the narrative, the conscious brain coming up with new options for the unconscious brain to mull overnight. The stories we tell ourselves are important, especially the ones that aren't true. The fairy tales, with magic and suffering and improbable yet happy endings; the fantasies of things we want to do; the endless replays of things we wish we hadn't. Sometimes the stories we tell ourselves are healing ones, stories that reframe the narrative, exploring it from an oblique place when the full story may be too much for us to bear. Sometimes the stories we tell ourselves allow us to make sense of things through repetition, the way Emi told and retold herself and me the story of Nate's accident, each retelling an act to free herself from the trauma of what she'd witnessed. But sometimes the most powerful stories we tell ourselves about ourselves are the bad ones, the ones we can't stop thinking about, the ones that wound us: the ones that say, *I'm always like this, this is always what happens, this is what I do, I always lose or fail or miss out or get left out or left behind.* Much of my parenting work involves talking my children through these stories, helping them learn to reframe them, to hear themselves when they say these stories out loud, asking them to examine those stories and question the reliability of the narrator to find out: What's the payoff for believing this particular story right now? What's in it for me to believe the story I'm telling myself?

Nate calls this "telling myself the bad story," and we work together to catch that kind of self-talk when it happens, attempting to recognize the moment when we are caught in the process of telling ourselves a story about what's happening in order to avoid the real story of what's happening, and then attempting to refrain from allowing ourselves to get lost in that story. It's tricky, and it doesn't always work; but even if they continue to listen to the story they've been telling themselves, the process of acknowledging for even a moment that it is, in fact, just one story, one way out of an infinite number of ways of interpreting things, helps them free themselves, just a little, from becoming stuck in the narrative.

It's not lost on me that my daytime work with them was work I continued to struggle with myself in the night. Why did I seem to need to keep telling myself this same story? What was my payoff?

What was I getting from this nightly narrative of blame, guilt, and fear, other than an extra helping of more blame, guilt, and fear? Why did I need to keep telling myself the bad story?

Before any of this, before the fever, before the ill-advised decision to leave the house and go out for breakfast, before the cough, I was in therapy, trying to come to grips with the realization that my marriage was over, that the thing I least wanted to confront was in fact the thing I must confront. Even though my therapist had known me for almost fifteen years at that point, for almost the entire length of my marriage, she asked me to tell her the origin story of my marriage and how I got to where I was then, at the point of its dissolution.

"But isn't telling you this story—telling myself this story—just a way to make this all seem inevitable? Make myself feel better?" I asked. "Like a 'just-so' story to justify everything, since now that I know how this is supposed to end, I can emphasize the foreshadowing, all the things I should have seen as warnings, reassure myself with a telling that makes this all a thing foretold?"

But she just smiled and said, "Humor me."

So I did. Eventually I was able to see that in urging me to trace back the story to its beginning, she wasn't trying to make me justify its end, but instead to create a different kind of narrative for myself than the one in which I found myself stuck. To find an alternative to the bad story I told myself about how I had failed, how I had finally done so badly at a thing it couldn't be undone, how finally the worst-case scenario of my being unmasked as a fraud and terrible person had come to pass. Retelling the story of my marriage to her, even though I knew it was an exercise, was a way for me to find a new story. And even if that story seemed to me to be false, by asking me to give it as much weight and consideration as other potentially false narratives about that relationship, she invited me to call into question the validity of every story I'd ever told myself about it, and confront the possibility that there could, in fact, be more than one way to frame things. In retelling her the story of my marriage, in creating a new story about how I got to where I was, I was able to be kinder to both myself and my then-husband, more generous to both of us, more forgiving. And by the time I was done with the process of retelling things from the beginning, I felt something besides the yawning free fall of failure: I felt compassion. For him, for our children, for myself.

I'm reminded of this process as I try to trace back the origins of this leak, trying to find some kind of narrative, some series of reasons or theories or explanations to make it easier to accept. And yet even as I know the importance of at least attempting to make sense of things, I can't shake the sense that in this case it is merely an exercise. Even if I could find my way back to the beginning of everything, find a way to explain it and make it all fit, organized and satisfying to the primal follow-through part of my brain that aches for completion, for order, it wouldn't change where I am now, or make it better, or undo it, or go back in time to prevent this unraveling. There is no story I could tell myself, I told myself, that could possibly change the facts.

But I continued to try. I tried doing what the man on the podcast did, tried to free myself from the tyranny of the bad story, tried to tell myself a new story with a happy ending. In this new story, I imagined the opposite of everything I'd done: I didn't send the kids away that weekend. Instead, Nate and I were sick together, spending lazy days in bed with the flu, and everything was fine. Or: Nate didn't get sick in the first place, and I didn't get sick either, and I didn't leave the house, I didn't cough, I didn't do anything out of the ordinary; I had a nice, normal, pleasant, uneventful weekend with the kids, and that was it. Or: I'd spent the weekend by myself and had an ordinary day and everything was fine. I imagined count-less different unremarkable scenarios, substituting the memories of ordinary days or the fantasies of normal, boring weekends for the facts of what actually happened.

It helped, a little, to imagine a different series of events, a story that didn't end with me messing everything up somehow, and being trapped in bed for nine months, in pain, unable to think clearly. But changing the story for myself didn't make the night terrors go away, no matter how many times I tried to revise the story into the story of an ordinary day.

Perhaps that was the problem, though: I kept saying "ordinary," encouraging myself to imagine that day as being an ordinary day instead of the day it turned out to be.

But the truth is, it *was* an absolutely ordinary day.

Because this is what happens on ordinary days. People make plans for the weekend with their children, or by themselves, on ordinary days. They leave their houses, or they stay inside, on ordinary days. They get married, or they get divorced, on ordinary days. They have heart attacks or strokes or twist their ankles or get bit by a dog or scratched by a cat or they fall down the stairs or get hit by a car or mugged by a guy on a bike who snatches their phone out of their hands. Or they narrowly miss hitting the car in front of them, or they stop themselves from tripping just in time, or they witness an accident and, miraculously, emerge unscathed. Or they don't; they get shot by a stray bullet, or killed by an angry ex-lover, or stabbed in a bar fight. They die in their sleep, or while playing catch with their kids, or with their family around their bedside, or utterly alone. These are ordinary days. We know this, we know that planes fly into buildings on spectacularly sunny mornings, that bombs are dropped on balmy nights, that floods creep and hurricanes rage and tornados sweep their destructive paths and then vanish on perfectly ordinary days. And yet we are lulled into this fantasy that a normal day is a day when nothing happens, while in actuality everything happens, all the time, and that is the reality of this life, that none of us gets out of it alive, and that every day we stay here is in fact the miracle, the unusual event, the aberration.

What happened to me happened on an ordinary day. I coughed, and something invisible tore, and that is a more ordinary story than a story about how all the millions of things that needed to go right in order for my body to exist as a functioning, healthy body moving through the world unimpeded and unimperiled did go right and everything was fine.

I don't know which story is more comforting: the story of a day when I imagined nothing bad or remarkable happening, or the story of a day when the bad thing that happened was, in the scheme of things, unremarkable. Inevitable. A simple fact in the midst of thousands of other facts that made up the story of that day, or any day before, or any day that might follow.

The content of my night terrors seemed like such obvious metaphors, they were barely even metaphors. They were direct statements from my brain, saying *You did this, this calamity is your fault*. It seemed barely worth interrogating, for what other meaning could it hold besides the one so overtly presented? And yet changing the story for myself didn't fully banish them; I still found myself waking up mid-apocalypse, playing out the same scenario. It seemed, like with Emi and her toddler grief, there was some kind of fundamental loss my sleeping self was struggling to process, something I was searching for outside of the phantom medication or gas mask or prepared plan that perpetually eluded me in my dreams.

Perhaps it was reassurance that I craved, I reasoned, some sort of logical refutation of the worries of unpreparedness that characterized my night terrors. Perhaps the story I needed involved pointing out to myself the things I had done to mitigate the real-life calamities of divorce and illness, perhaps that would be enough to soothe the primal me that was tormented in the night. And so I tried reassuring myself before going to sleep, speaking to myself out loud, explicitly reminding myself: *You did everything you could, you prepared for everything, there's nothing you left undone or unattended to, you've done everything you needed to do.* Sometimes it would be a general benediction; other times I would run down a list of concrete actions I had taken, or things I had done.

This helped, but, again, not enough.

One night, going through my litany of reassuring self-talk, trying to figure out what part of the story I was missing, I stopped for a moment and just lay in bed, listening to the sounds around me, feeling my breath, feeling the way it felt to be in my body. I heard cars going by, buses in the distance, the muffled conversation of people walking past my house on their way to a restaurant or bar or home, the sounds of the city at night. It was the soundscape of the past year or so of my life, lying in this bed. For some reason, recognizing this moved me, and I felt myself beginning to tear up. These ordinary sounds were the soundtrack of my own helplessness. Stuck in bed, unable to get up without pain, unable to stop this thing happening inside my own body, or fix this thing that was somehow broken; this was the background sound of hopelessness, of the frustration of feeling responsible for what was happening and yet utterly incapable of fixing it. Somehow it made sense to me that this was connected to the night terrors, this fear and horror and blame, and I had the sudden notion that what I needed in this moment was not my nighttime list of reassurances that I'd done everything I could do, not a note to myself reminding me what was real, not a soundtrack of relaxing delta waves.

I'd begun telling myself a better story, but what I needed wasn't just a different narrative. What I needed was the thing I found when retelling the story of my marriage. What I needed was compassion.

What I needed was *forgiveness*.

Not me telling myself: *You did everything you could.*

But instead, me realizing: *There's nothing you could have done.*

Who would expect the end of the world to strike in the dead of night, vines descending from the ceiling to strangle you, expert assassins with deadly lasers to slice through your walls, poison gas to seep in through your vents, a chemical attack requiring protective medicine or at least an antidote?

No one, because those things are ridiculous. Un-anticipatable. Unrealistic. Unlikely outside of a nonsensical, very bad disaster movie. No one could prepare for those scenarios, or, better yet, prevent them, because they are virtually impossible.

And who would expect that coughing due to an illness, a tickle in your throat, swallowing the wind, or just because you have to cough would cause a tear in the fabric of your reality? Who would prepare for the likelihood of their dura tearing from a nearly involuntary reaction to throat irritation that millions of people around the world, right at this moment, are experiencing in the form of an everyday, ordinary cough?

No one. No one would anticipate that. I could not have anticipated that.

I didn't have to keep holding myself accountable for failing to prepare for a thing that I didn't even know could happen.

There's nothing you could have done, I told myself. *Nothing.*

And even though it wasn't exactly a fairy-tale ending to the story I'd been trying to tell myself for so many months, for the first time in a long time, I slept all the way through till morning.

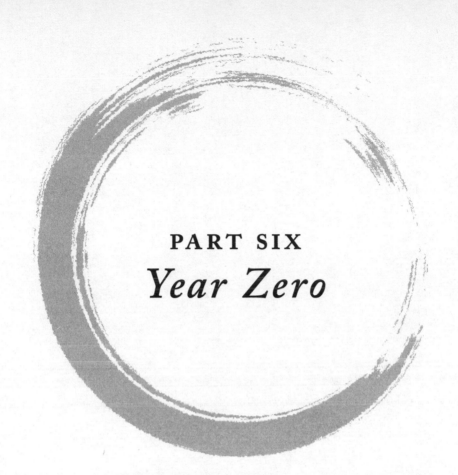

PART SIX
Year Zero

"I have tried to explain over and over again how mind changes brain structure and function, but nobody alive has yet properly defined mind and no one has explained properly how so-called ethereal thought can change so-called material structure. The whole subject is filled with wonder."

—Dr. Norman Doidge, as quoted in
The Guardian, February 8, 2015, "Norman Doidge:
The Man Teaching Us to Change Our Minds"

34

April 2016

W ords are still difficult. Reading too many in a row makes my brain hurt, exhausts me. But I'm able to tolerate it better now. I find myself slowly returning to the pleasure of reading paragraphs at a time before I must nap to recoup my ability to perceive, to read, to understand, to think in metaphor and simile, to hold concepts in my mind. Writing is harder: Sometimes I can think of a thing, even imagine how it might make sense on the page, on the computer screen, but by the time I get there, language is an impossible mystery. I cannot translate the wordless thoughts in my head into English. Even the thought of trying to explain what I am thinking becomes overwhelming, and I must rest and try again later.

I go into stores now and I remember why I'm there, but the brightness and volume still overpower me. I feel my brain reject the totality of the stimuli around me, feel the gravity of my thoughts sinking into some solid form, coalescing, cementing, becoming impossible to process. I can feel the place where my thinking is done shut itself down like a snail pulling itself back into its shell. Loud people and places assault my brain, and even on a calm day, my best cognitive self is limited in time: It exists from whenever I wake up in the morning until about three in the afternoon, when I begin to flag, when my brain surrenders to the fog, to the rebound headache pain I still grapple with. I need lots of sleep. Not as much as I did right after my procedure, when I slept twelve, fourteen hours at a time, and still napped during the day, but more sleep than I ever used to need. By three o'clock each day I feel my brain slowing and have to lie down; by five o'clock each day, I have roused myself for the process of going through the motions of preparing dinner and supervising homework, desperate for release; and by 7 P.M. I am asleep.

All of this is progress, though. I remember two weeks after the procedure, when Dr. Kranz called to check in on me and follow up, I had a cumulative daily upright time of four hours, total, and was still fluctuating between what felt like leak headache pain and what felt like high-pressure pain. He'd said that was normal, that I should gradually increase my activity level and upright time, if I was able; that I should track my progress so as to note patterns and reassure myself by being able to look at a bigger picture of overall trends instead of just the day-to-day experience, which could seem disheartening. I have done this, I have tracked my symptoms, I have quantified my days, I have tried to take the long view and be patient. Three months post-procedure, I can manage four hours of consecutive upright time and seven hours of cumulative upright time on a good day. At our most recent check-in, Dr. Kranz reassures me that time will continue to be my friend; that he is confident, from what I've described to him, that my symptoms will continue to improve; that he is optimistic I'll be able to get back to normal; and that I should try to continue to take things one day at a time and focus on the progress I've made over the past few months.

I have hit many small milestones. Some are physical, like sitting with my children through dinner; attending parent-teacher conferences and surviving the conversation, being able to think and talk and respond without becoming overwhelmed, even though it takes me a day of rest to recover; walking the mile and back to pick up the kids from school. Some are internal, invisible victories. Remembering a PIN code for the ten seconds it takes me to view it on my phone and then enter it on my computer. Being able to read a chapter of something and remember what it was about, have it linger in my mind and make sense, resonate with some other ideas. Watching short television shows on my iPad, in bed, without becoming overwhelmed by the sheer amount of information happening at me, light and sound and smash cuts and musical cues and dialogue and expression. I feel my brain slowly waking up, like a limb that's been asleep, prickling and heavy with the feeling of sand.

Once I'm able to read more and retain information, I find myself craving stories of explorers. I read books and listen to podcasts about adventurers, both ancient and modern, coming to grips with the limits and capability of the human brain and what is required of it to function. I learn about what happens to brains at high altitudes without oxygen; about monks who light up fMRI machines as they regulate their body temperature and meditate their human bodies into submission. I read about people who travel to Antarctica on missions, some foolhardy, some scientific, and the madness of cold and sensory deprivation. About mountain climbers compelled to risk their lives and push their brains to their limits, sometimes suffering the same kinds of symptoms as people with intracranial pressure problems, strokes, brain injuries. About shipwrecks and crashes, about poorly planned trips and failed expeditions. About the mysteries of illness and the body, the mysteries of health and the body, and the quest for understanding the brain and mind and how they work with the body in the context of health and illness.

Part of why I think I feel so drawn to these stories of explorers, so compelled to read them and listen to them, is that I myself don't have a map. My recovery process is uncharted territory, my view of the way forward as limited as the infinite whiteness of a snowstorm on the Antarctic tundra. The doctors treating spinal CSF leaks are only beginning to understand the true mechanisms of injury and how to repair it, and most information pertaining to recovery is focused on the immediate physical experience of healing from repair procedures and avoiding recurrence of any leaks. And if there is a paucity of research on spinal CSF leaks and their effective treatment, there is little to no research at all on what happens to the brain while cerebrospinal fluid is leaking, or what happens to the brain in the aftermath of having had a spinal leak. I was given instructions to follow when I went home in terms of my physical recovery—no bending, no twisting, no lifting, limited caffeine and salt, the practical-life accommodations I must make—but no instruction at all for how to help my brain recover, other than to just rest and give it time, wait it out. And so I am drawn to these stories of people who mapped out previously unmapped places, who set out to explore places no humans had been before and mark the path for others, who were also trying to survive in parts unknown, with limited guidance, if any.

As part of my instinctive quest for stories, for ways to understand the ways that the brain protects itself and heals from injury, I also listen to neuroscience podcasts and read books about the plasticity of the brain, and the ways in which the brain is able to adapt and change in response to behavior, even in the case of severe trauma.

I learn that, contrary to what science used to teach us, the brain does not become a fixed and unchangeable thing after childhood, and that in fact it is capable of growth and change and reorganization—what neuroscientists call "neuroplasticity"—throughout all of life, even well into adulthood. Brains are resilient.

One book in particular, *The Brain's Way of Healing*, by the Canadian psychiatrist Norman Doidge, offers a fascinating look into the history of medical thinking about the brain and how our concept of the brain has changed as we've learned more about it, and how thinking of the brain as a thing capable of change has opened up new ways of understanding and treating brains injured by stroke or concussion or other trauma. He writes of patients with Parkinson's, chronic pain, dementia, multiple sclerosis, traumatic brain injury, epilepsy, stroke, all able to modulate their symptoms through a range of techniques designed to encourage the brain's natural capacity for change. Some of these techniques I am familiar with, like biofeedback (using information you receive about your body's functions to learn to control those functions—one example of this is when a patient is hooked up to a sensor that displays their heart rate, allowing the patient to see the difference that is made by breathing faster or slower, and thus to learn to lower their heart rate on their own); others involve specialized medical devices still in development or not otherwise available to the general public. But much of the research seemed to point to focused, small, physical movements requiring intense concentration—such as practical-life exercises, like using a stroke-impaired hand to stack cups or wipe countertops—as being the most useful thing for patients suffering brain damage due to illness, trauma, or stroke.

In the book *Soft-Wired: How the New Science of Brain Plasticity Can Change Your Life*, Dr. Michael Merzenich discusses the circumstances under which the brain's natural neuroplasticity can be harnessed to create focused neurological change. One important factor he notes is that change is more likely to take place in a brain that is prepared to take advantage of it. Being engaged and motivated helps prep the brain, neurochemically, for learning and change. Being distracted and merely going through the motions of something without making much effort doesn't require a high level of engagement, and thus the brain doesn't "pay attention" to the opportunity for change. In addition, the more focused and alert a person is on the task at hand, the greater the possibility of change. And since part of what is changing when you are focused on mastering a task and engaged in the process is the strengthening of connections between neurons working together, the more you practice and work at whatever task you're focusing on, the more those strengthened connections become lasting change. This cooperation between neurons also helps the brain become able to rely on those newly established connections, and be able to better understand and predict patterns, anticipating what comes next.

Change, of course, in the beginning, in almost any context, is temporary: Doing something once doesn't ensure that you've learned it forever, no matter how alert or engaged you are. Change becomes permanent through repetition, and also, somewhat contradictorily, through novelty. So part of making change happen is doing a thing over and over while finding ways to focus and concentrate and renew your engagement each time, so that your brain finds the experience novel enough to make it a part of your permanent record, rather than just a temporary file. Remarkably, this repetition doesn't always have to be physical: The brain can be changed by imagining and rehearsing something mentally, without moving the body at all. Memory helps reinforce learning, and mental rehearsal of something new helps reinforce that change, making it become more permanent. And interestingly, for the damaged brain, every moment of new learning is a moment that helps the brain stabilize itself. As new neuronal connections are made stronger through mastery of new skills, other neuronal connections are weakened—including those neurons whose indiscriminate firing contributes to the issues brain-injured people can have with information overload, sensory strain, and executive function. Learning new skills in a focused way can help create new neuronal connections, strengthen neuronal pathways, and calm neuronal overactivity.

When stroke patients consistently performed and practiced concentrated, focused activities, such as using an arm weakened or impaired by stroke to stack blocks or wipe a table or pick up small objects, researchers noted not only physical improvements in terms of fine motor skill control or greater stamina or strength. They also noted improvements in speech and memory and other cognitive deficits. Somehow, their brains were able to make new connections, find new ways around the places damaged by stroke, find new ways to adapt and to heal, just from this intense, challenging, task-based work.

I read all of this—slowly, resting when necessary—with great interest. Because, just as in the stories of explorers, I recognize myself in some of the descriptions I read about patients struggling with brain injury. I didn't suffer a stroke or a trauma due to concussion or whiplash or brain lesion or other neurological issue; but I recognize myself in the symptoms many of these patients describe in the aftermath of their illnesses or accidents as they recover. The way their brains are overwhelmed by sounds and visual patterns. The way that they only have so much brain energy per day, and the way that means their brain function declines as the day goes on. The way their short-term memory fails. The way words sometimes elude them, or become confused with one another, homophones interchanging themselves, or become entangled, rhyming and repeating, mesmerized by sound instead of meaning. The way social interactions fatigue them. The way narrative is a challenge.

But the other reason I find this all so interesting, reading through it with my healing brain as I wait through the purgatory of physically healing without knowing for sure if I'll start leaking again, is that it reminds me of something. The physicality of small, focused movements; the repetition of these movements, with the brain at full concentration; the mental rehearsal of these movements; making these movements seem new and exciting, all in the service of learning a new skill, forging new neural pathways: All of this reminds me of work I did with my children when they were toddlers, building things and stacking things and playing repetitive games to nourish their growing brains. But even more than that, it reminds me of the work I have done ever since I was eight years old; work I did sometimes for upward of six hours a day, every day; work that likely helped wire my growing brain in the first place.

It reminds me of practicing piano.

35

The room was grand: dark wood paneling, enriched with details from floor to ceiling, carved patterns that repeated themselves throughout the room; tall windows flanked by thick, heavy curtains, with sills big enough for a person to sit and peer into the courtyard below, mournfully, after a bad lesson; high ceilings; rug-carpeted floors. Two Steinways, side by side, one for the student, one for the teacher.

Mrs. Kim introduced herself, holding out her hand. It was fierce—the handshake, the hand itself, with its veins and knuckles and muscles; and her surety, her firmness, her sense of gravity. My hand felt especially pale and formless and small in hers. I was seventeen. She was probably younger than I am now, but to me then she seemed ageless, beyond age, beyond any concept of aging.

"I remember your audition." Her voice was heavily accented, hard to understand. She was barely taller than I was, but she was imposing, her movements fluid but controlled as she released my hand and walked to the set of pianos in the middle of the room, her steps light but centered, like a ballet dancer's. Everything she did seemed to have a sense of purpose.

"I remember your Mozart. And some Liszt? Fiery," she said, allowing an eyebrow to raise, a small hint of a smile. I wasn't sure I understood what she was saying, and it must have been clear on my face, because she clarified for me. "You like the quick. The dazzle."

I did? But I nodded my head.

"Refresh my memory," she said, languidly gesturing to the piano. "The Liszt."

I nodded my head again and sat on the padded bench. I hadn't practiced the Liszt in months; the summer before leaving for music school I had mostly spent my time waitressing, saving money. There hadn't been much time for practice—at least not at the level I'd been practicing before, while preparing for competitions and music school auditions.

I began the piece, trying to get a feel for the piano, the pedal, the ease of the keyboard as I went along. I realized too late I had started too softly, and now my pianissimo had nowhere to go. I tripped on some of the faster figurations and I could feel my cheeks flushing, the cycle beginning of my own awareness of my mistakes informing my performance, making me even more likely to make mistakes, making me hyperaware of how many mistakes I was making, leading to more mistakes, and on and on and on.

Suddenly she stopped me, a strong hand on my right forearm.

"That's fine," she said, but this time there was no eyebrow raised, no hint of a smile. "We have a lot of work to do."

Two days later I was in a third-floor practice room, crying. I could hear the sounds of everyone else practicing around me—Mozart from down the hall, Bach, Beethoven; the room next door to me thundered with sounds I'd never heard from a piano before. I paused to listen, feeling the vibrations of an octave bass passage reverberate through the floor.

I turned back to my music. A Chopin étude. After listening to me play barely a minute or so of Liszt, Mrs. Kim had already made up her mind: I was to learn this étude—but not the whole étude. I was to return next week having practiced just one note.

The first note.

Of only the right-hand part.

For a whole week, that was all I was supposed to play.

She told me I should "strike from knuckle, not wrist." I should "feel belly button here," in that one finger, as it rested on the note, so that that one finger was the center of my body. And I should do that, over and over, until it sounded right. What did that even mean? I couldn't tell. It all sounded the same to me. It sounded embarrassing. Like punishment. Like failure. One week at music school and I was relegated to playing only one note, like some kind of beginner.

I wiped my eyes and then wiped my hands on my jeans. Screw it: I had played this one stupid G-flat for twenty minutes, trying to strike from my knuckle, trying to make my third finger my belly button, whatever that meant, and all that had done was prove that it was possible to play one damn note for twenty minutes. I launched into the Lizst that she hadn't liked, playing too loudly, using too much pedal.

This piano felt easy, the action quick, the keys responsive, the room bright with sound. It was easy to be loud, to sound full and powerful and accomplished. One note. Was she kidding me? I reached the first cadenza and trilled a decrescendo of alternating chords into the quietest pianississimo I could manage in the small, echoey practice room and felt chills as my hands hovered above the keys, a muddle of pedaled harmonies fading away as I waited through the fermata. Then I dove back in, playing the theme again, this time an even more elaborate incarnation. My tempo was skittish, the pace quicker than the way I usually played it, and I went with it, chasing it through the cadenzas and the flourishes and the triumphant, final iteration of the theme, through the crashing, flashy coda, finally, to the end, with a majestic last chord, the kind of ending you imagine when you imagine a concert pianist ending a piece, flushed with sweat, almost standing up from the bench to make that final chord sound the way it needs to sound, one hand up in the air after the last note, waiting for the audience to stand and cheer and fill the moment with the sound of raucous applause.

My moment was filled with the ambient silence of the practice room, plus the sounds from the other practice rooms: opera singers, pianists, clarinetists, violinists, all rehearsing at once. Reality.

I sat there in the muted cacophony of the practice room noise, letting everyone else's practice sounds wash over me, and returned to the score. Chopin. G-flat. One note.

"Think like squirrel," she told me, the next week. "You know squirrel? They run, they move so fast, quick—and then they stop. Very still. So still, nothing moves. They conserve energy."

I played the G-flat with my third finger, trying to strike from the knuckle, have my belly button there, think like a squirrel.

"No," she said, batting my hand away. She demonstrated, her powerful hand striking the key in a way that sounded different from the sound that I'd made. "Be totally still. Then play. Then still."

I tried again.

"Like squirrel," she reminded me. "They don't fall asleep."

Of course squirrels fall asleep, I wanted to argue, but I thought I knew what she meant. The way they freeze and yet aren't frozen with tension, the way they are able to be still without ever seeming sloppy, relaxed. Was that what I was supposed to do? Play a note and then freeze in time, my hand stuck in a position but without stress or tension? Had I been playing the note and then letting my hand relax too much, when what she wanted me to do was basically play a one-note, one-person game of freeze-tag?

I tried again. G-flat, third finger, strike from knuckle, belly button here, think like squirrel, don't fall asleep.

"Yes!" She said. "Again!"

I tried again, doing everything exactly as I did before.

"No," she frowned. "Tension in fingertip only."

I tried again, G-flat, third finger, strike from knuckle, belly button, squirrel, don't fall asleep, tension in fingertip.

"Better," she said, but her face was stern.

The so-called Black-Key Étude, nicknamed for the fact that much of the melody is played solely on the black keys of the piano, begins on a G-flat, third finger, right hand. The third fingertip is the center of your body. All the gravity is there. The third fingertip strikes the G-flat, wrist and palm moving in protectively, and waits. You should be able to lift yourself like a gymnast and balance on that centimeter of flesh. The sound bells, rounds, becomes flat, fades away. You do not move. You breathe. You feel the gravity.

Your hand should look the way it looks when you drop it loosely to your side: wrist relaxed, the plane to your knuckles a natural forty-five degrees or so, your fingers curved, the blood settling into your fingertips. That is where the gravity is, there, in the blood. The trick is lifting your hand to the keys while your mind imagines the hand is still dangling beside you, your shoulders loose, your neck relaxed, no tension.

Though the G-flat sound has died, you are still there, hand crouched in position, balancing around that third finger. You are not moving, but you are preparing. Then quick, like one of the squirrels in the park, motionless until it moves: your fifth finger to the B-flat. If you have not prepared properly, your knuckle will collapse. Make it strong. Now the center of gravity is your pinky. Someone watching but not hearing you will not be able to tell the difference between the way your hand looked when you played the G-flat and the way it looks now. Your hand is cupped, fingers huddled around one another, but not gripping, not tight; it should appear as though if you turned your hand palm up, keeping it in the exact same position, you might be cradling a baby chick.

The point is to strike and then be at rest. That is why the energy, the tension, must be concentrated in the fingertip, why the rest of your hand—the rest of your body—must remain neutral, balanced, supportive. Slow practice is about preparation. In slow practice you learn to conserve energy so that at tempo you have the stamina to support your speed.

The B-flat has sounded, rounded, and died while you rested, alert, upon the key. Next is D-flat, your thumb. It's easy to misuse gravity with your thumb, easy to make a harsh tone using the same force that had elicited a rounded one with your pinky. Your thumb has more natural weight, more natural gravity behind it. The trick here is to play decisively but not crassly, and this time you attack with the side of the appendage and not its tip, the black key against your thumb from its tip to the first joint, the rest of your hand returning to its default position, resting, relaxing, preparing.

Those are the first three notes.

Eventually, after practicing like this, deliberately, thoughtfully, in slow motion, one note, then two notes, then three, then enough so that the first phrase was executed and the next part was just a repeating of the pattern, I was allowed to think about my other hand, the left hand accompaniment. Eventually, I was allowed to put them together. Eventually, after weeks of painstaking, focused work, I was able to hear the difference between the sound Mrs. Kim wanted me to make and the sound I actually made, was able to feel the difference between the way Mrs. Kim wanted my hand to be and the way my hand actually was. Eventually, I was able to play the piece at speed, in all its fiery, quick dazzle, and while I didn't understand exactly what it was I was doing all the time, or whether I was doing it the way she wanted me to, I began to understand there was a way to think about playing music that was different from the way I'd thought about it before. At tempo, the étude was hyperspeed, fingers blurring through virtuosic passages, sounding light and effortless, dancing on the keys. But it only got there through the slow, deliberate, intentional work of slow, deliberate, intentional practice.

In the end, I was thwarted by the showmanship of the last measures, a double-octave black key scale before the final cadence of the piece. My small hands weren't able to wrap around those octaves, no matter how much slow work I did, no matter how much resting and preparing was built into the practicing of it. There are some physical limitations even smart practice can't solve. But this exercise in patience, in approach, in practice, laid the groundwork for me for the rest of my time with Mrs. Kim, and the rest of my life as a musician.

Later I would learn how the work doesn't end once you gain a new understanding of it. How once you're able to play it through without snagging on difficulty or tugging the thread too tightly, the next stage begins. How you must allow yourself some perspective. How you must recognize the ways in which the piece has changed from your deconstruction of it—that slow, deliberate practice. How you must reimagine it in its new context. How you must attempt even newer ways of understanding it.

How you must take it apart again.

Left-hand only, to even out the bass, to comprehend the way it grounds the melody in this particular piece but perhaps not another; to dissolve the rest of it away until only the skeleton of the structure is there, guiding you toward another way of listening.

Right-hand only, the voicing, the phrasing you thought was one long breath but is actually several groups of thoughts in this particular piece but perhaps not in another; hearing now so clearly how in isolation the information this melody imparts is completely different than what is conveyed when it is integrated, grounded by harmony and structure and form.

Then how you must put it together again. Right and left, with this new understanding.

And take it apart.

And put it together.

And take it apart.

How you must perform it as though you are discovering it all as you go, inventing it right at this very moment as the perfect expression of what you might say if you only had words to express it.

And how later, when you have truly forgotten, when the piece has fallen out of your hands and ears and mind from lack of practice, you go back to the beginning and start again.

36

I don't start with one note, like the one my teacher had relegated me to in my first weeks at the conservatory, but I do start at the beginning, with the most basic part of being at the piano: sitting.

Although my dura is no longer as sensitive as it was in the early weeks after my procedure, when slumping or having my chin down even slightly provided immediate, painful feedback that my posture should be corrected, at four months out, it is still sensitive enough that sitting for any length of time gives me a near immediate headache. The dural sac extends past the end of the spinal cord, and sitting creates a kind of compression of this sac and the fluid within it. Normally this would have no effect at all, and yet now, with my brain so sensitized to changes in pressure, with the nociceptive fibers innervating my dura so alert for potentially damaging stimuli, and ever at the ready to translate that information to my spinal cord and brain as pain, as danger, I feel the consequences of sitting almost as instantaneously as I would the stubbing of a toe. My intracranial pressure increases, and the headache begins, bringing with it the attendant brain fog and nausea. Unlike the pain of a toe stub, however, this high-pressure headache and brain fog can take hours to subside. My hope is that sitting at the piano, which requires the kind of posture most favorable to the dura and spine, will help me tolerate the side effects of sitting down, and that any playing I will do will function as both a distraction from the pain and, not incidentally, as a kind of occupational therapy for my brain.

Sitting at the piano is its own exercise, as it is the base for proper technique. You must sit with your weight distributed evenly, neither to the left nor the right, your feet resting, also equally weighted, on the floor. Your spine should be elongated, as though there is a string attached to the very top of your head, toward the back of your skull, pulling you slightly upward. Your shoulders are down, relaxed. Your arms are at your sides, relaxed. When you bring your arms up, when you bring your hands to the keys, your shoulders should remain down and relaxed, which is the tricky part. But a relaxed shoulder is crucial: Your relaxed, elongated spine and your relaxed shoulders and arms are the conduits for all the energy and tension that should end up in your fingertips, not stuck in a slumped back or hunched shoulders or tense wrists. Your arms are like wings, joined at the center point between your shoulder blades, emanating outward, your fingertips light as feathers.

The center point between my shoulder blades is, of course, where my leak was. And so sitting in a way most beneficial to my dura is especially crucial as I bring my arms to the keys and attempt to play. Every sound I make at the piano has its physical starting place in the muscles and nerves around the site where I was torn, and though there is something satisfying, even poetic about the thought of this, the thought of music emanating from a broken place, there is also an element of danger: I don't want to stress the still-healing area too much, I don't want to strain the sensitive spot. And so I sit, upright yet relaxed, and bring my hands to the keyboard imagining a line of energy that flows from the leak spot, energy leaking out toward my shoulders, down my upper arms, past the potential stopping places of my elbows, of my wrists, and all the way to my fingertips, unimpeded.

I don't start with one note, but I do start small. I think about what I learned in my reading about patients recovering from traumatic brain injury, the importance of those small, focused, repetitive practical-life tasks in their healing process. It was the smallness of them, the level of concentration required, the repetition of them, that seemed to help the brain find new ways of thinking, of rewiring itself, of making new connections in places where the old connections were broken seemingly beyond repair.

And so I start with a book of Pischna technique drills, a set of sixty progressive exercises that are purported to help with finger independence—the ability to control each finger independently, without tension or interference from nearby fingers. (This sounds like an easy task, fingers working independently; but place your hand on a flat surface in front of you and try to lift each finger one by one, without the other fingers moving. The thumb and index finger should be relatively easy, perhaps even the third and pinkie fingers, too. But that fourth finger: lifting it up without your other fingers joining in for moral support is tricky, and even if you can do it a little bit, it's almost impossible to lift it as high as you did your index finger, for example. This is due to the ways in which the muscles tangle in the back of your hand, and depend upon each other. As a pianist, it's important to work against that codependence and try, as much as possible, to untangle that knot.) These exercises require concentration, relaxation, coordination, and repetition. In other words, they seem to be a perfect fit for what I'm hoping to accomplish with this homegrown brain-rehab therapy.

Even something small, like this, is a challenge for the brain. Playing these exercises requires the use of both hands, which involves coordination between and cooperation by both hemispheres of the brain. Looking at the score while playing the music requires eye-hand coordination, and also involves the mental task of translating marks on a page representing tones into their proper embodiment of sound via the correct keys on the keyboard. To know whether or not I have succeeded in the effective translation of these printed notes into their corresponding audible notes, I have to be able to listen and hear and evaluate and, if necessary, correct and respond. There is auditory feedback, visual feedback, physical, muscular feedback, left-brain/right-brain feedback: so many levels of engagement required of the brain, just to perform the simplest, most basic exercise in the book.

I begin with just ten or fifteen minutes per day, starting with these Pischna exercises. The early ones are basically short phrases built off a pattern of one or two notes of a chord being sustained while an upper melody vacillates between two notes, first moving back and forth from one note to the note above it, then between the top note and a note just a half-step above that. Then the pattern is repeated a half-step higher, and so on and so on, until you have repeated the full pattern on every note of the chromatic scale. I remember doing these exercises in my early days at the conservatory and becoming quickly bored by them—*Yes, okay, I get it, it's a pattern, whatever*; I much preferred my teacher's main technique of making technical exercises out of tricky passages in whatever repertoire I was trying to learn. But now, focusing on trying to sit in such a way as to align my spine and not aggravate my dura, focusing on getting these small, precise finger movements right, it feels like a challenge, and my brain feels soothed by the melodic pattern rather than bored by it. It provokes a feeling in my brain like the tranquil puzzle games I played while stuck in bed, leaking, the same games I play now, while listening to podcasts, recovering. It's the feeling of things fitting into place, the satisfaction of patterns fulfilling expectations. It makes my brain feel full, nourished.

When I was leaking, and enveloped in brain fog, playing piano was both a reassurance and an exercise in implicit memory. Explicit memory is the kind of memory you use when you recall an anecdote, or remember an event that happened to you, or do anything that requires a conscious effort in retrieving information. Implicit memory is the kind of memory you use when you don't have to think about anything at all: brushing your teeth, washing your face, tying your shoes. Implicit memory doesn't require conscious, executive control. Implicit memory is what enabled me to walk to the store to run an errand; my CSF leak–induced problems with explicit memory were what prevented me from remembering what I was supposed to buy when I got there. Sitting at the piano and playing through old repertoire when I was leaking involved implicit memory, the muscle memory of years of practice from years before, and it was soothing to be able to play, to know that a part of me was still there, remembering things, able to do some things, even if my executive functioning brain was not explicit enough in its instructions to follow through on others. This new piano therapy I've devised is forcing the use of both implicit and explicit memory: the implicit muscle memory of having done these exercises, however haphazardly, at some point in my past studies; and the explicit memory of doing them now, remembering what I discover and learn as I go through the process of doing them now, and applying that knowledge moving forward, whether in the next moment or the next measure, or on the next page or the next day.

I begin to gradually increase my practice time, from ten or fifteen minutes to a full half hour, as my tolerance for sitting increases, and soon I begin to increase my musical scope as well, moving from technique exercises to scales and arpeggios, to the comfortable muscle memory of old repertoire. I find my music books from when I was in high school, and begin to read through pieces I learned when I was thirteen, fourteen, fifteen. I recognize my old teacher's handwriting on the page, indicating tempo, cautioning about problem areas, underlining tricky passages. And more than that, I recognize memories, as I play through these pieces. Most practice sessions over the course of a musician's life do not involve the kind of high-level focused concentration I'm attempting now—sure, there is focus, and sure, there is concentration, but when you're practicing six to eight hours per day, it's just not practical or even possible to be on high alert the entire time. I spent many hours in practice rooms thinking about breakfast while playing Brahms, or letting my mind wander as I meandered through some Mendelssohn, supplying my own off-topic narrative to his Songs Without Words. Playing through this old repertoire from high school—Debussy's First Arabesque, Scarlatti sonatas, the third movement of the Beethoven Pathetique, which I learned one year for the annual Sonata Competition—I not only remembered the pieces themselves and how they felt in my fingers, I remembered the feeling of practicing them, in some cases, specific thoughts I had working on specific measures on a specific day at a specific moment in my practice time. It was as though in awakening those neural pathways, I gained access to memories that had been long buried there, and were now able to be uncovered, like the snow melting away after months of winter and revealing the sidewalk underneath, along with everything that had been there when the snow first fell. This happened as I moved on through my old repertoire, too: playing through one of the middle-years Beethoven sonatas I'd learned during my first year of music school, I remembered not only the slightly terrifying memory that had always stayed with me, of

Mrs. Kim standing behind me in the third-floor practice room where we were, for some reason, having a lesson that day, and physically provoking me, prodding me, pushing my back, poking me with her strong fingers to startle me into a forte sound during an octave passage that was difficult for me to reach; but I also remembered the memory of practicing the page before that passage, and being able to hear the person in the practice room next door practicing the Chopin Fourth Ballade, and thinking about the way the light was coming in through the window to my right, and the way the trees were starting to regain their leaves again, and about how soon I would be able to take a break and knock on the door next door, and wondering if he could hear me as clearly as I could hear him, and whether or not my small hands would be ultimately too small for this piece, wondering whether in the end it would defeat me, but also wondering what I might have for lunch, and whether I might go over to his house later, and whether he still loved me. All of this came back to me, all at once, a full paragraph of memory, as I played past that measure, and I marveled at all of this information stored somewhere deep in my brain, and wondered how much else was there, buried and otherwise inaccessible, waiting for the snow to thaw.

Within a month of starting this practice, I begin to experience the feeling of my brain reconnecting itself, like going from dim Fourth of July sparklers of ideas to full-on fireworks. It reminds me of the way I felt on the table during my blood patch, or during the CT myelogram at Duke, when after being injected with fluid, I felt the fog lift and my mind become clear, when I felt myself become Me again. I'm still struggling with regaining my explicit memory, with things like executive function and organization; I still lose words and find myself overwhelmed by situations which previous to all of this would have been trivial for me to handle. But a month into this piano therapy, I am able to hold ideas in my head, to remember numbers and dates, to have moments of insight. I can make connections between concepts, I can remember things better from one moment to the next, complete tasks more efficiently, have wide-ranging conversations and not lose my train of thought. Is this happening because of this piano practicing? Is it because I have more than twenty-five years of music training already in my brain, ready to be reactivated? Would other people without previous training have similar results?

It makes me curious: Is there a difference between learning new music I haven't studied before now versus revisiting repertoire I learned and spent hours practicing as a teen, a time when the brain undergoes remarkable and significant development? Is there a difference between reactivating old pathways versus creating new ones? Or is my brain different now, after this leak, so that even those old pathways, from those decades-old years of practicing, when reactivated, become like new?

It also makes me curious about the idea of the self, about how the self that is me now recognizes the thoughts and memories of the self that was me when I first learned the piece of music I'm now revisiting. About how the self that was me when I was leaking felt cut off from the self that was there, lost in the fog, the "real me" that emerged when I had a bolus of fluid injected into me, raising my intracranial pressure, and—somehow—allowing my mind to once again resurface from the depths of my brain.

I think, too, about my experience of illness during those years in music school, when I battled with some of these same questions: the questions of pain, of being believed, of the value of my own narrative, of who I was. When I was sick then, with what I called Mystery Disease, and in the years afterward, when I recovered, I'd thought of that time as partitioned off, compartmentalized from the rest of my life. That was not the Real Me; that time I spent being sick was some kind of strange exception to the rule, some kind of secret side-quest, some deviation from the norm, not the Real Me, the me who was ordinarily healthy and productive. That compartmentalizing, I came to understand, was a choice I made to protect myself. My experience of myself as a sick person didn't make sense with my experience of myself as a well person; it didn't cohere. So thus it couldn't be truly me. It was an aberration, a time in my life that was the exception, not the rule.

But before the leak happened, back when I was reading through my journals from music school while working on a book idea about conservatory life, I was suddenly able to see the continuity. That sick, struggling self in those journals, writing about being sick and not wanting to be sick—that self was still *me*. I recognized it. I saw it in the attempts at narrative, at understanding. In the stitching up of story, in the denial of story. I saw it in the comments written in the margins from Future Me's at later times in my life, now all of them Past Me's, evaluating what I'd written, taking issue with things, revising, correcting, reevaluating, clarifying, discounting, admitting. Reading through these diaries, this writing from a me who was at the time only slightly older than my daughter is now, I was able to accept and genuinely embrace, for possibly the first time in my life, a coherence of self. I was still me, even then. That sick me, that lost me, that ashamed me: *It was still me.* I was able to recognize it now. It was me, even when I thought it wasn't, even when I didn't want it to be. Sick me was actual me, is present me.

It was fitting, in a way, to have stumbled upon that self-acceptance, this understanding of continuity and coherence of self, before the CSF leak happened. Because although my experience of the leak was in many ways an experience of dissociation, of a splitting off of implicit me and explicit me, a distance between brain and mind, a sense of selflessness, I'm able to understand that I don't have to understand this illness and recovery as a period of being Not-Me. I don't have to decide now, the way I decided as a teen, as a young person in my twenties, to discard the time I spent lost and sick as Not-Me Time, some kind of distraction from Actual Me, all of it a Me that didn't count. This CSF leak took my sense of Me-ness away for a time, and now, as I recover, I'm reintegrating, relearning what it's like to be me, right now, in the midst of a process. Recovery is putting the pieces back together. Just like in piano practice. The part after you take everything apart, and do the slow, careful practice of putting it back together; the part after the deconstruction.

The entire self is a story we tell ourselves without even realizing it. Like music, the self assembles in real time. Moments are stitched together to make a seamless whole. Reactions moment to moment assemble a personality, a behavior, a summary of self. We think of a melody or a symphony or a song or a self as one solid thing, when it's just this and this and this and this, finite moments pretending to be infinite.

The more I practice piano, the more I invoke the coordination of sight and sound and concentration and memory and physical motion and intellectual analysis, the more I feel my brain return to itself. The more I am able to understand that perception is a fiction the brain is constantly creating. That our seemingly intact, seamless experience of consciousness is actually a series of discrete moments we stitch together so quickly we're not even aware we're doing it, creating movies out of still pictures, solid substance out of fluid particles, progression out of stasis, cohesive self out of individual, unconnected moments. That I assemble myself as surely as the way a series of notes tricks a listener into hearing what sounds like a song.

Part of what's been puzzling me throughout this whole experience is the very question that puzzled the doctors at its inception: *When did this start?* And so I've been endlessly tracing my steps, as if locating that moment was the key that could unlock the door to all explanation. But at a certain point it doesn't matter anymore where you started; at a certain point, it only matters where you are now, and where you go from here.

Of course, when you're performing a piece of music, especially for other people, it does matter where you start. There must be a context. It doesn't make sense to begin a piece in the midst of the middle development section of a sonata, or initiate listeners with the bonus content of a coda, the tail end of a piece. Playing music is just like telling a story: You begin at the beginning, and let everything else follow from there. This allows the listener the opportunity to understand how the entire piece unfolds from the smallest of gestures at the very start, how the first measures hold the clues to everything—structure, melody, shape, intent. Everything is there, if they are able to listen, if you are able to lead them to it as a performer. If it works, they will understand, even if what they understand is not your own specific understanding.

But when you're practicing it doesn't matter where you start. In fact, it's better to start anywhere but the beginning. The more you can deprive yourself of context, the more you are able to fully pay attention to the work. Start at the end and work backward. Isolate the difficult measures of a secondary theme. Transform the dazzling, flashy, fast passage into a technical exercise, break down the cadenza, mirror your right hand with your left to understand the finger work, work in dotted rhythms, work at half tempo, work at the slowest tempo possible. Look at it all inside-out. Don't allow yourself to be lulled into the story—unless, of course, it is the moment in your practice when you must be lulled, to understand what work is still left for you to do.

Practice is the back of a needlepoint, all tangled threads and chaotic stitching. Performance is the front, the pleasing picture whose existence depends entirely upon that messy hidden work. It's the process, the daily practice, the work nobody sees, the hidden music, that makes performance possible.

Illness is the back of a needlepoint, all tangled threads and chaotic stitching. Full recovery is the front, the pleasing picture whose existence depends entirely upon that messy hidden work.

I'm not performing yet. I am somewhere in between the chaos and the finish. I am recovering. And so I can start anywhere. I don't need to know where the beginning is, I don't have to determine where it might be, I don't have to choose a precise moment when it all started, and when it all went wrong. Because in practicing, it doesn't matter, and the more I practice, the more I see that in life it doesn't matter, either. I pick a point, and work from there, and that's the work, that's the point. Every day I work a little longer, increase my stamina, nourish my brain, and every day it helps me stop the futile quest for the answers to everything, which of course could never be located in one perfect, precise moment. Every day I continue to start where I am, because I'm not performing, not yet. I'm practicing.

37

June 2016

B y early June, I have been practicing my piano brain therapy for almost two months, and when I check in with my doctors, they all ask me the same thing: "What the heck have you been doing?" My therapist and my neurologists note my improved facility with words, my improved ability to make connections, to understand concepts; my improved ability to have insight and to be able to express that insight, my improved ability to follow complex instructions and remember things. They notice my boost in executive function, my increasing ability to tolerate noise and other sensory information, my overall improvement in general. "Are you taking any new medication?" they ask me, and I tell them, excitedly, "No, this is my brain on music." I share with them the findings of this highly-selective, ultra-biased, one-person ongoing research study I'm performing, and while they're skeptical of its true efficacy, not to mention its replication possibilities, they're happy to encourage me to keep going. "If it's helping you feel better, keep doing it," they tell me.

So I do. I try to spend forty-five minutes each day practicing piano, helping my brain get better, helping my dura increase its tolerance for sitting. At the point when I feel a sense of diminishing returns—when the playing becomes easier, when I notice my mind wandering instead of concentrating—I try to mix it up: sight-read unfamiliar repertoire, work on learning a piece that's totally new to me, take a familiar piece of music and break it down so that I tackle it in small chunks starting at the end of the piece and working my way to the beginning. I try to fool my brain by taking things out of context, now that my brain is getting better at understanding context. I try to focus on both repetition and novelty, to encourage my brain's ability to change, to reorganize itself, to heal.

By early June, it is also nearly six months since my procedure at Duke. The six-month mark has been a milestone looming so far in the future it seemed a myth. When I was leaking, time wasn't a concept I could fully participate in. I couldn't think in hours or days, couldn't make plans for the next week or month; I could only exist in moments, one minute to the next, everything disconnected, discrete. In the beginning days and weeks after being patched, it was still difficult to think ahead, to project myself to a point in time beyond where I was at whatever moment I existed in at the time, because healing was still so new, so fragile, so time-dependent. When I began to feel better, when I began to improve, I began to have a better sense of what I was capable of—I could plan to take a shower knowing I would need a nap afterward; I could plan to be upright, walking around for an hour, knowing I would need to spend a corresponding hour lying down, recovering. And eventually, I could make plans a day in advance, a week in advance. It no longer seemed like an impossibility to think about the future and rely on the fact that I'd probably be able to be a part of it. I could make a plan for a faraway time and assume I might be okay by then, maybe even better than I was when I made the plan in the first place.

But it feels like tempting fate to think about meeting that six-month mark, the unit of time Dr. Kranz said it would take for me to know whether or not I was past the most tentative, risky part of healing from my patch. If I can make it to the six-month mark without the leak recurring, there's a very good chance it might not recur at all. I'll still have to hold my breath to make it to the one-year mark, when the chance of my spinal CSF leak re-leaking would be even smaller; but making it to six months without the leak coming back would be a very encouraging indication that my prognosis is good.

Still, it feels risky to hope.

"'Hope' is the thing with feathers," begins one of my favorite Emily Dickinson poems, and right now I understand it, the small bird you hold in your hand, the lightness of it, the fragility, its fleeting nature, the possibility that, at any moment, it could fly away.

In the leaker group, I read posts from people who were patched months before me who never made it to their six-month mark, who began leaking again days or weeks after returning home. I read posts from people who were patched after me who are already leaking again. Occasionally there are encouraging posts from those former leakers who are "sealed and healed," in the terminology of the support group, and back to living full lives comparable to how they lived before their leaks began; but most of the posts are about grappling with pain, with the uncertainty of whether or not a leak has truly been fixed, with the disappointment and grief of having a blood patch fail, of having a surgery fail, of having everything fail.

My best friend from the leaker group, Nina, the funny, upbeat former lawyer who went to Duke two weeks after I did, has been my patch partner, my partner in recovery. We check in with each other daily, comparing symptoms, commiserating with each other about the awfulness of rebound high-pressure symptoms, reassuring each other when those symptoms subside and seem to be replaced by the old familiar leak symptoms. We make jokes about the medical realities of our lives now, the torture of sitting, the annoying, unyielding slope of the wedge pillow we hope to one day never again have to use. We dream about the day we are both free of headaches, rebound or otherwise, when we can have our lives back. "But this *is* our life right now," she reminds me. "We're not waiting, we're in Year Zero, the year we start over."

But as we get closer to that six-month mark, our paths begin to diverge. I'm experiencing far more high-pressure days than leak-feeling days, with the majority of my symptoms being due to the effects of a higher intracranial pressure than I'm used to; and she's experiencing more leak-symptom days. No longer is she needing to sleep on a wedge pillow to prop her head up, and no longer do caffeine and salt make her headache worse. Lying totally flat now is what makes her head feel better, and caffeine and salt either do nothing, or ameliorate her pain slightly. She's back to having only minutes of upright time before the headache comes on, looming into sensation at the back of her head. "I'm leaking again," she tells me, "I know it"; but I don't want to believe it. She has been suffering with her spinal CSF leak for so long, far longer than I suffered with mine. She's been leaking for nearly a decade, she's had multiple surgeries. She deserves to recover more than I do.

"Don't be ridiculous," she says when I tell her this, but it doesn't feel ridiculous to feel guilty. I want us both to sail past the six-month mark, to fly through the eight-month mark, the ten-month mark, all the way to the end of Year Zero and the beginning of

Year One, the year we will be past the bulk of the healing process, with all of this, hopefully, behind us. I want this for everyone who posts in the leaker group, for everyone who tells stories about jobs lost and marriages broken, about missed diagnoses and botched surgeries, about setbacks and complications, and losing all hope.

The last line of the Emily Dickinson poem says of hope, this feathered thing, that "Yet—never—in Extremity / It asked a crumb—of me." And it may be true that hope asks nothing of us. But it feels sometimes like hope is a lot to ask for in the first place. For the people on the board who are still suffering, for people like Nina, hope seems like nothing but crumbs, and it doesn't seem fair for me or anyone else to hoard them. I feel a gnawing survivor's guilt, as pressing and real as the fear of relapse.

Even if I do make it to the six-month mark without leaking, there's still the chance that I could start leaking again at any time; it's just that the chance is smaller. The uncertainty is still there, no matter what milestones I hit. "You can do it," Nina tells me. But I'm not sure. I hope she's right, and yet I don't want her to be right, because I don't want to do it without her, I don't want to do it if it means leaving her behind. I don't want that to be how the story ends, for either of us.

Endings are tricky, though. How will we ever know when this is over? Is there a point at which we can truly stop worrying about relapsing? We have both spent countless hours trying to trace our way back to our beginnings, attempting to find the source, the starting place where it all went wrong; and we have both come to understand the folly of thinking that there could be one moment that changed everything, even if we could find it. Endings seem to be as futile as beginnings: just as difficult to find, maybe even impossible to pinpoint, and equally beyond our control.

I keep practicing piano, starting at the beginning and playing through to the end, starting at the end and working my way through back to the beginning. I keep thinking of how a piece of music is a closed system, like the central nervous system, like the dura that encases my brain and spinal cord, and of the variability and fluidity that's contained within it. I keep thinking about time and how repetition helps my brain, and how practicing is all about repetition, and how even in repetition there is variation.

There's an old music joke: *How do you get to Carnegie Hall?* The punchline, of course, being *Practice, practice, practice.* It's not exactly funny (in the way that older jokes aren't always funny to modern ears), and it's not exactly true (in the way that practice alone isn't a guarantee of high-level artistic proficiency)—but there is a piece of truth built into the joke, and the clue is in the repetition of the punchline. *Practice, practice, practice.*

Practicing piano is all about practicing repetition and expecting new results. Playing scales and arpeggios over and over, solidifying movements into muscle memory. Breaking down patterns, recognizing patterns, repeating them to make music physically easier to play, easier to understand. The very idea of music itself is built on repetition: repetition of melodies, of phrases, of chord progressions. Repetition is even built into the musical structure of a piece, ideas iterated and reiterated. From the sonata form of exposition, development, recapitulation—taking a theme, developing it, and placing it in different contexts, making it all the more meaningful and savory when the theme returns, repeated in its original form—to the verse-chorus-verse-chorus-bridge-chorus structure of contemporary pop songs. It's all about repetition.

There is another joke about repetition, doing the same thing over and over and expecting new results. The punchline to that one, however, is that that is the definition of insanity.

But I keep moving forward, keep practicing, keep repeating, keep tracking my symptoms, keep checking in with Nina and hoping against hope that we can meet our six-month mark together, our brains foggy with sealed-up pressure instead of leakiness. "This is the goal," Nina reminds me. "To get better. It's fine if you get there first. You can do it for both of us." But I want to bring her with me, to the other side of the six-month mountain, where we can rest together after the high-pressure climb to the summit, never to repeat it.

38

There are several things leakers live in fear of after having their spinal CSF leaks patched, all of which are made more terrifying by the fact that these fear-inducing things are actually all normal, everyday occurrences. Everyday life becomes fraught with tension, infused with the low-level anxiety of a horror movie, as we try to move gingerly through the world without disturbing the patches, awakening the beast, restarting the leak. I dread the prospect of a summer cold, fear the consequences of a sneeze, under no circumstance do I ever want to find myself in the grips of a coughing fit. I worry about bending forward too forcefully, about twisting too hard, about running, about jumping, about falling.

I have been lucky thus far to avoid the school-borne colds and bugs my children bring home with them—"It's nothing personal," I tell them, as I slowly back away, avoiding their hugs, moving myself out of the line of fire of their coughs and sneezes, "I just never want to cough again ever in my entire life. You guys get it." But then one morning while walking down the stairs, mere weeks before hitting my six-month, no-leaking milestone, my luck runs out: I slip on one of the top steps and fall hard, landing with my full weight on my right hip before tumbling down the other ten stairs and coming to rest on the landing. Nothing is broken, thankfully; but the bruises blossom immediately, and all I can think is: *I've ruined it I've torn the patches. I'm going to start leaking again.*

I lie down with ice packs on my back, my butt, my knee, my arm where I caught myself on the banister during the fall, and I take some Tylenol for the pain. I'm supposed to take the kids to their grandparents for the day, but my skin hurts when I walk, and my muscles cramp from the assault. I put on compression shorts under my summer dress, even though I know they will squeeze me, squeeze my dura and make my brain foggy with an upward push of fluid, but the compression helps contain the sensation of the growing bruises, so I make the trade-off. I sit on the train gently, balanced on my left leg and butt cheek, since the right one is so tender, and every jostle makes me wonder if this is it, if I've torn open the leak spot, if all my recovery has been for nothing.

The pain from the fall at first is almost welcome, because of how different it is from the kind of pain I've become so used to. It's almost a relief to experience pain that's not a headache, pain that has a different kind of immediacy and texture to it. And yet somehow, after a few hours, it starts to feel as though this pain from the fall has become the gateway pain to all the other pain in my body that has been holding itself at bay, waiting for the right time to manifest: I feel the ache of my arms, my ankles, my back, the nagging, worrying throb of a wisdom tooth beginning to emerge.

By the time we arrive at the grandparents' house, when I check on my bruise I'm horrified to see it is already a massive red and purple welt covering my entire right butt cheek, and my jaw ache begins to morph from an annoying nagging sensation to an insistent stab. I lie down with ice packs on my butt and Orajel on my wisdom tooth, which has picked the absolute worst time to try to break free, and say to myself over and over, *Please don't let me be leaking again, please don't let me be leaking again,* a pathetic incantation that might as well be a leaker's prayer.

I commiserate with the other leakers, posting about my fall, my hurting tooth, my worries that I might have undone my almost six months of progress. I tell Nina about my fall, about how my butt hurts, about how bad the bruise is, about how I can't even tell if I have a leak headache because of how bad my tooth pain has suddenly become. As my bruises deepen and spread, it becomes impossible to lie on my back or my side, and I have to somehow sleep on my stomach while keeping both my butt and my head elevated, which seems as comical as it does impossible. The bruise darkens to a horrifying purple-black and I try to sleep with a heating pad on my butt as I lie in a constellation of pillows, googling things like *ass bruise death* and *wisdom-tooth pain death* and *can falling down stairs give you a spinal CSF leak* and *can a person die from a really bad butt bruise.*

A part of me keeps thinking *Why, why did this have to happen, why did I have to ruin everything when I was so close to being out of the woods? Why am I back, stuck in bed again?* Part of me keeps replaying the moment of the slip, the feeling of the wooden stair sliding from beneath the arch of my foot. Will this be the moment in time I will return to, hoping to undo by sheer repetition of thought, as the start of some new leak, or aggravation of the old one? But another part of me remembers what my piano teacher always said, about rest being an opportunity to prepare. *You hurry, hurry,* she'd told me. *But there is time. Feel it.* I have been hurrying, hurrying. This fall is forcing me to slow down, is giving me an opportunity to take the rest I need, to feel time instead of rushing past it.

If the defining feature of my nine months in bed with a spinal CSF leak was isolation and existential doubt, the focus of my nearly six months of recovery so far has been the strangeness of moving between the realms of the sick and the well. It's not a linear progression, and even on the days when I have moments in which I can pass as being better, I'm not fully recovered, not yet. Every day I monitor my symptoms, scanning for clues that can tell me whether I'm healing or leaking again, whether I'm mending or tearing, whether I'll have my life back or be back to being flat on my back in bed for life. What I'm learning as I recover is that recovering means forgetting, thinking I'm better than I really am, pushing myself to do more, tolerate more, force myself to forget I'm not healed so that I can force, in a sense, the inner work of healing. But falling down this flight of stairs reminds me I'm not ready to forget just yet. I should not be forgetting to acknowledge my need for carefulness, my need for rest. I should not be forgetting to honor the importance of small victories like sitting up all the way through a movie, or experiencing a few hours without a headache, or lasting an entire day without taking a nap. I still have more healing to do. I am not performance-ready. There is still more practicing to be done.

Remarkably, this ungraceful tumble down the stairs has bruised my ego and my butt, but not my spine. I move toward meeting my six-month milestone with bruises along a spectrum of deep purple to a nauseating yellow, but with no leak, or at least no leak symptoms. My wisdom tooth decides it has had enough, and tries to escape my head, the pain of which feels like a kidney stone in my jaw and reduces me to tears. Those old pain-scale questions from the headache center now suddenly have a true context: I have found my 10/10 pain, my worst can't-go-on-living pain, and I gain a new respect for my old leak headache, which felt awful and omnipresent, but at least had the common decency to only ever reach a 9 at its worst. I have the tooth extracted, a process I've been fearing and putting off for years, and I sit tentatively, almost hovering in the dentist's chair, my butt tender from bruising, my head on fire from tooth nerve pain, my neck and spine anxious to prevent flexion or stress on my dura. Afterward I'm given instructions to follow once I get home to care for the wound site, and these instructions are so thrillingly straightforward, so incredibly practical, so amazingly limited in time and scope, it is a true relief. I'm almost excited to go through this particular healing process, which at no point will involve any fear whatsoever that coughing or sneezing or bending wrong or falling down the stairs will cause my tooth to grow back and hurt me again.

My friend Nina's path continues to diverge from mine. She suffers no fall down the stairs, no rogue tooth requiring extraction, and yet her slide back into leaking symptoms continues unabated. By the time of her six-month milestone, she is almost 100 percent certain she is leaking again. All of her high-pressure symptoms are gone, and the rhythms of her life have returned to what they were when she was leaking. The headache a heavy weight at the back of her skull, the fatigue and exhaustion and pain upon standing, the tinnitus and blurry vision, the brain fog. "It is what it is," she tells me. "At least it's better than being in that awful rebound high pressure. At least I know what to do when I'm leaking. That's a comfort, at least."

∽

In July, a month after Emi turns 17, as I meet that six-month milestone, she and I take a trip together, the first big, sustained thing I have been able to plan and manage in over a year. She has just finished her junior year of school and is beginning the process of applying to college. She's decided she wants to go to art school, and her top choices are Parsons, at The New School, in New York City, and the Rhode Island School of Design, in Providence, Rhode Island. She'll be doing a three-week summer school program at Parsons, living on campus and taking classes, a kind of mini college experience, during the last three weeks of July. And so we decide to take a trip up to RISD the week before that, over the Fourth of July weekend, to tour the school and visit friends in the area. It is just Emi and me, the two of us having a bonding weekend together. It reminds me of the weekend she'd suggested we have after Nate's accident, how she longed for some time together, just us, to help us heal from the trauma. This trip is also serving a healing purpose, the two of us connecting again, just us, in the aftermath of a different kind of traumatic experience.

We are traveling by train from Philadelphia to Providence, which means five hours of sitting, a marathon of sitting, the most sitting I have ever done at this point in my recovery. I plan accordingly. I bring my ice turbans and a travel pillow, plus a special angled pillow to sit on to help my back. I plan to take breaks, to stand up and walk the train aisles when sitting gets to be too much. I take a rolling suitcase Emi will be able to lift for me if necessary. I pack the medicines I might need: a diuretic my neurologist has recommended, to help with the high-pressure headaches I'm still dealing with; some lorazepam in case of sensory overload.

Traveling is stressful. I'd underestimated how much of my recovery and progress has been dependent upon the predictability and calmness of my daily routine at home. Here, out in the world, with so much new input, both visual and aural, my brain strains under the weight of so much heavy lifting. I find myself exhausted and overwhelmed, trying to put a brave face on it for Emi while also trying to find places to rest. But we manage to have fun, shopping in the deserted downtown mall, every place a ghost town due to the holiday weekend; laughing over trash TV and comedies at the hotel; gossiping over her social group's summertime social media habits. We go to the school tour, and I stand through the introductory session, as I have had my fill of sitting after the marathon train ride. Emi and I both stand out: me due to my being the only person standing up, provoking confused looks from other parents, who gesture to open chairs as an offering for me to sit down; and Emi due to her hot-pink hair. I'd expected more startling hair colors at an art school campus tour, but so far we've only run into a few other kids with bold hair choices: turquoise, royal blue, a faded purple strand here and there.

We follow the group we're assigned to on the tour, and the campus is beautiful, a tiny town of classroom buildings. Everything that is described to us about the course of study and the opportunities for students sounds amazing to me, and I keep nudging Emi like *This is fantastic, right?* But as the tour goes on, and we walk from un-airconditioned building to un-airconditioned building in the hot sun, we both begin to feel ourselves flagging. We sit down at one point, while the rest of the group explores a classroom, and I ask, "What do you think? Pretty incredible, yeah?" And she half-smiles and says, "Yeah, I don't know. It's awesome, but it's not in a city. I think I might want to be in a city. Like, a *real* city."

As the tour group is led across a green space that is touted as some kind of social gathering spot, Emi leans on my shoulder. "Wanna get out of here?" I say, and she immediately agrees. She's hungry and thirsty; I'm tired and need to lie down. So we loiter behind the rest of the group until we are free to break off and go our own way unnoticed. We find a restaurant nearby and get some food and drink. The restaurant is set up so that the tables are next to deep, long, built-in benches, stacked thick with cushions. I'm so tempted to lie down, and Emi says, "Just do it! You're exhausted!" So I ask the server if it's okay if I lie down on the bench for a minute and she looks at me like I'm crazy for even asking and tells me to go for it. We eat our lunch and I lie on the bench, propped up with pillows, recuperating before we head back out into the sun and find a taxi to return us to the hotel.

The next night we visit friends for dinner, friends we've known since Emi was twelve or thirteen, who live nearby. I rest all day so I can be ready for the noise of teenagers excited to reconnect and catch up in person, plus the competing din of grown-up dinner table conversation, and once we get there, it is a comfort to see them. I've explained a little, via email, about what's been going on with me, and with our family, over the past year or so, and so it's not so hard to talk about. I've also become better at being a narrator, about understanding which details are important and which are irrelevant to what a listener wants to know, about being able to tell my story, our story, without saying more than I need to or more than someone is ready to hear. I'm grounded in a timeline now—the flu, the cough, the pain, the diagnosis, the treatment, the halfway point, the prognosis— rather than lost in a muddle of context-free facts and feelings and uncertainty. And things aren't as raw, as new, as painful. I can talk about the divorce as a matter-of-fact thing, about all of it as a matter-of-fact thing, and it all feels, if not understandable, at least able to be understood.

We end our trip by traveling back through Boston, where we are able to spend time with one of my aunts and with my grandmother, Emi's great-grandmother. Nina, my leaker friend, lives outside of Boston, and I threaten to meet up with her, too, but she says no, I shouldn't bother adding another leg of travel to this already big trip. "When we meet, it's going to be when we are both fully sealed and healed," she tells me, "that's the plan!" Her daughter also went to art school, to RISD, in fact, and now lives and works in fashion in New York City, and Nina's other plan is for us to meet her when Emi goes to the summer program at Parsons. And we do: Barely recovered from our big trip to Providence and Boston, I travel with Emi to Parsons a week later, to set her up for her three-week summer school course, and we have lunch with Nina's daughter, Nina Skyping in from bed to say hi. "Next time we do this, we'll all be there in person," Nina says, and I concur.

Emi thrives at the Parsons summer session, finding her way in to understanding and expressing her experience of the last year and a half of upheaval in her life through a photography project she undertakes. Her anxiety series of photos captures the claustrophobic, dissociative feeling of panic attacks and disintegration, and she has a breakthrough, not just in finding a new way to process everything she's been feeling, but in transforming those very personal feelings into something artistic and universal. She, too, is becoming better at mastering a narrative, at learning how to tell the story of her life. Her photos provide a context, an entry point for understanding, a way in. She's no longer just taking pictures. She's making sense of a process. She's making sense of herself. She's making art.

In the fall, after school resumes, when she's in the thick of the college application process, I take her to National Portfolio Day, where representatives from all the major art schools across the country come to a city and evaluate the portfolios of prospective art school applicants. She meets with reps from six schools, including

Parsons, and all of them are impressed by her anxiety series. All of them mention her excellent use of light, of perspective; her remarkable understanding of how to center herself in the dramatic moment, to frame a scene; the cinematic sensibility she brings to her photos. She speaks with the Parsons rep longest of all, maybe forty-five minutes of critique, and comes away from the experience feeling heartened by the feedback she receives. She adjusts her portfolio, tailoring each submission to the comments she received from the school representatives she spoke with at the event, and finishes her applications far ahead of deadline. She has decided, after her summer experience there and the great feedback she got from the rep at National Portfolio Day, that Parsons is her top choice, and she submits her application early, even though she's not applying for early decision. And yet, within weeks she is noti-fied that she is accepted along with the early decision applicants, and is awarded a generous scholarship. Her voice on the phone when she calls me from school is shaky, filled with wonderment and disbelief. She's done it: She's in. Her top choice chose her. My voice is shaky, too, filled with pride, filled with gratefulness to see her begin to emerge on the other side of this awful period of uncertainty.

I think about how resilient she is, how strong her instincts have always been. I shared with her once that Camus quote, about how "In the midst of winter, I found there was, within me, an invincible summer." It reminds me of her, how forceful she is, how capable she is of re-centering herself, even in times of upheaval. It makes me feel relieved, as a mother, to see the pure continuity of self in her, the way her impulses now to make art and heal are outgrowths of those same instincts she had as a kindergartener, as a grade-schooler, to grow toward the light. The Camus quote con-tinues: "And that makes me happy. For it says that no matter how hard the world pushes against me, within me, there's something stronger—something better, pushing right back." There is something strong inside me, pushing back, as I fight my way through this recovery; but it puts my heart at ease to know there's something even stronger inside her, able to push back against the world, no matter what it hands her.

39

September 2016

Even after passing my six-month milestone of recovery without leaking, I'm still plagued by cycles of rebound high pressure. Sometimes this seems linked to my menstrual cycle, with my headaches and pressure increasing the week just before my period arrives, and subsiding once it's over. But sometimes I feel stuck in a high-pressure vortex, my head squeezing tight behind my eyes, the part of my spine between my shoulder blades throbbing, with no relief, no matter how much dandelion tea I drink, or how long I wear the ice turban, or how much I avoid the things that trigger it (caffeine, salt, sitting). I notice that during these times, when it feels as though my high-pressure symptoms are as intense as they were in the days and weeks after patching, that my blood pressure is also high, and I wonder which thing is causing which. Is my high intracranial pressure causing an increase in my blood pressure? Is high blood pressure causing me to have symptoms of intracranial hypertension? Or is it some kind of cycle involving both systems, hypertension stoking hypertension?

For a while I battle this with diuretics, medications that make me pee every five minutes. This may clear out some fluid, but it doesn't do much else to help my symptoms. Eventually I'm prescribed some blood pressure medication. Perhaps lowering my borderline-high blood pressure will help lower my intracranial pressure as well.

Time is your friend, Dr. Kranz had told me, early on in the recovery process. And it's true that the passage of time has generated some proven results: I am older, my kids are older; my body and brain are more accommodating, and have more stamina; my cerebrospinal fluid production, while still evidently a little stuck in overcompensation mode from time to time, has calmed itself as the months have passed. Time has also helped in terms of understanding what has happened to me, what has happened to our family. There is a routine now, something predictable to depend on: I have a general timeline for healing and a place to go if the leak comes back; the kids have a schedule of when they're with me and when they're with their dad. We are becoming used to the new routine, the new prognosis, the way all kinds of inflamed, tender things are beginning to become soothed.

It's difficult to send my kids away, to pack them off for the weekend, and not think about the weekend I sent them away with their dad and ended up coughing myself into a spinal CSF leak. I worry, as I send them away, that there may be some other danger, and I worry, as I send them away, that I won't be there with them to help them deal with it. They are both angry, upset, lashing out more at their dad, who is a bigger target than I am right now. I'm sure my time will come, the time when they allow themselves the full expression of their sadness and grief and anger at me for having been sick; but for now the anger they wrestle with is wrestled with their dad, and my heart breaks thinking of them working through these things without me, fighting and standing up for themselves and setting boundaries and doing this hard work without me there to help them. Yet isn't this exactly the work they should be doing, regardless? Isn't this the work they would be doing even if I hadn't been sick, even if there were no divorce? At thirteen and sixteen, at fourteen and seventeen, shouldn't they be differentiating themselves from us, being angry or defiant, fighting for independence? Isn't that normal? Still, I sit with them as they come back from their weekends, teary-eyed about a fight or discussion, an inability to be heard, and I listen to them and soothe them and remind them that what they're doing is hard work, that I'm still here, that nothing bad happened to me while they were gone.

One weekend, though, in early September, when they're with their dad, a bad thing does happen. I take the blood pressure medication I've been prescribed, as I have for the past day or so, and after a little while, I begin to feel a heaviness in my chest, as though I can't breathe. I change positions, sitting up, because when I lie down, the heaviness and tightness in my chest is worse. I know what the signs of a heart attack are, and I know they can be especially subtle in women; but I think, *How ridiculous would it be for me to have a heart attack right now, when I've just taken blood pressure medicine?* I check my blood pressure and am surprised to find it to be very low. Wouldn't it be high if this were a heart attack? I wait it out a little bit longer, but my chest tightness and heaviness continues, and it becomes harder to breathe, and I begin to feel a weakness in my left arm. I begin to type *chest heaviness tightness arm* into Google, and before I can even finish, results are populating, all of which seem to be some version of *Get to a hospital, you're gonna die*. I know that Emi is planning to have a difficult conversation with her dad tonight, that she may need to talk to me afterward. But I don't think I can wait until then. I summon an Uber and direct it to the nearest emergency room, figuring that if this is nothing, they'll just send me home after my having successfully wasted everyone's time. But when I get there I discover two things: one, that telling the intake person at the ER "I think I might be having a heart attack" gets you bumped up to the very front of the line; and two, that it is not a waste of time.

According to the doctors, who look at the EKG results, I have had some kind of "ischemic event," meaning that the blood flow to part of my heart was constricted or restricted somehow. Not a heart attack, they don't think, but some kind of event that stopped enough blood from reaching my heart for a small period of time. It's possible this could be a rare reaction to the blood pressure medication, but they're not sure. They need to keep me overnight, monitor me to make sure it's not really a heart attack, and then have me evaluated by a cardiologist, who will do an echocardiogram and some other tests to see what's going on with my veins.

I'm moved from the ER to a room in the cardiac part of the hospital, where I'll stay overnight, and as I'm being hooked up to another EKG and examined by doctors, having my blood drawn and other tests performed, my phone starts blowing up. It's Emi: Her conversation with her dad hasn't gone well, and she needs to talk to me about it. She has sent dozens of texts and attempted at least five FaceTime calls. My phone is dying, nearly out of battery; and I also don't know what to tell her. I don't want her to worry. But my not responding is as worrisome to her as any response might be.

Finally, I text her. "Sorry," I say, "I can't talk right this second. Can you give me a few minutes?" But she can't wait, she's upset, she's crying, she's scared, she says, she needs to talk to me right now. So I tell her I really want to talk to her, but I can't right at this moment, and she demands to know why. Finally, I say: "The first thing you need to know is that I'm fine, I'm going to be fine. But I had a reaction to the blood pressure medicine I was taking, and I have to stay in the hospital overnight." I don't tell her I'm being evaluated for a heart attack, that right this very minute I'm covered with little stickers attached to electrodes, but it's still too much for her to take, and she calls me, crying. I talk to her for a few minutes, trying to calm her down, telling her I'll be able to listen to her tell me what happened in a little bit, when the doctors are done checking me out. Gil texts me, "How could you tell her you're in the hospital?! She's so upset right now!" And the doctors ask me, "So, have you been under any stress lately?"

I'm woken up throughout the night to have my vitals checked, and each time my blood pressure is very low—90 over 50, 100 over 60. In the morning I'm released from the hospital and sent to be evaluated by a cardiologist in the next building. He listens to my story, examines me, looks at my test results from yesterday and overnight. I tell him about my experience with spinal CSF leak, and where I am in my recovery process, and the cardiac nurse perks up: She has had a CSF leak herself, not once, but two times, both due to a faulty epidural during childbirth. Hers resolved fairly easily, though she did have to have a few blood patches with the second one. We're both excited to talk about our shared experience with leaking, but the cardiologist isn't sure my CSF leak has anything to do with what's happened with my heart. My echocardiogram is normal, my stress test is normal, my stress-echo (where they perform a stress test and then do an immediate echocardiogram right as you hit your peak exertion point) was normal. "Everything looks great," the cardiologist says, pointing out my strong arteries, my non-obstructed veins. It doesn't make sense to him that this could all be due to a reaction to medication, but he tells me not to take the medicine anymore just in case, and in fact cautions me to not take anything at all besides aspirin. This could be pericarditis, he says, an inflammation of the sac around the heart. "What is it with me and sacs of things in my body not working right," I attempt to joke; but again, he doesn't think what's going on has any relation to my leak. And then I'm free to go. I should take aspirin for three months and follow up with him sometime after that. Maybe we'll try another blood pressure medication; maybe not. Until then, I should just take aspirin and try to minimize stress. "Tell that to my kids," I say, but it really is just a joke. They're doing their best. They're recovering too.

Between my fall and this strange response to medication, and my waxing and waning high-pressure symptoms, my recovery feels very much plagued by setbacks, events that cancel out any progress I've made. It's frustrating: I'd thought that once I'd passed the six-month mark, it would be smooth sailing, or at least a steady progression of improvement, no more zigzagging through a series of progressions and relapses. But that's not how this goes, I'm learning. Nothing about this process is easy or predictable. It's messy, it's inefficient, it's uncertain; it's human.

Practicing piano helps my brain feel a little more in control of a process, breaking things down and building things up again, raveling and unraveling, performing exercises to solidify a skill, but working in such a way as to be able to take advantage of a spontaneous moment, to try something new. Beginning to write again is more daunting: I can write in small bursts, but I have to think about it a lot before and after; editing, a thing I used to be able to do as easily as playing a Beethoven sonata, is another thing that now must be reduced to its component parts in order for me to understand it. I write a little, and then, instead of being able to edit what I've written on-screen, or even mark it up on a page, I have to print it out and cut it up, make each sentence mobile, manipulable, able to be physically moved around in space so that I can better understand it in the context of time, of succession. When I confess this technique to a writer friend, she laughs at me: "That's literally how I work!" Still, it is strange to me that things that used to make sense as purely invisible thoughts and ideas now only feel real and understandable when they are physical, palpable things I can manipulate with my body instead of my mind. But I try to adapt: I print things out and cut them out and move them around and retype them, and, just as with my piano practice, it does get easier.

I recommit myself to taking things slow again, recommit myself to the slow practice of sinking into my life and taking my time, doing the physical things I need to do to get well, allowing myself the mental space to continue waiting things out, growing stronger, getting better, getting my systems circulating again the way they're supposed to. Reestablishing a rhythm with my kids, allowing them the relief of seeing me improve and reassuring them on the bad days that this is how it goes: slowly, and not in a straight line. This helps them, too, I think, knowing that slow progress is still progress, that they're okay, too, that things are happening even when it seems like nothing's changing. That part of the process of this, of all of this, from my illness to their adjustment to our new family configuration, is acknowledging the meandering nature of growth, its natural mystery.

My friend Nina's mystery is also beginning to be uncovered: After months of decline after our post-patching paths diverged, the reason for her recurring leak is becoming clear. She returns to her neurosurgeon in Boston, who had performed a previous surgery on her spine, and when he goes in to look for the source of her continuing spinal leak issues, he discovers something he'd never previously encountered in a patient before: a rogue blood vessel, shooting out of a nerve root sleeve in her spine, shunting cerebrospinal fluid away from where it should be and sending it into her circulatory system. She was leaking due to what's called a CSF venous fistula, an abnormal channel between the space where cerebrospinal fluid is and a vein outside the dura. This is something difficult to see on imaging; and yet it explained why in her case the numerous blood patches she'd had had done nothing to seal her up. Because the problem, in her case, wasn't a tear or a leak. It was her own body, siphoning off cerebrospinal fluid through a vein. She has this vein repaired, tied off so that it can no longer redirect cerebrospinal fluid away from where it circulates within the dura, and now she waits. Her Year Zero clock is reset, beginning again, restarting her recovery, just as I'm about to begin my own personal Year One.

40

I am an unreliable narrator.
In truth, I always have been. I know this now.

Long before my brain became a fish out of water, long before my cerebrospinal fluid slowly began to seep away through a tear somewhere along my spine, I understood in a general sense that there were moments when I was fooling myself, talking myself into a story to force my life to make more sense, adjusting that story when it butted up against subtle but inconvenient points of reality, revising that story into a tidy narrative that worked, even if it wasn't exactly one hundred per cent true.

Even in those times when my life seemed to hand me a story ready-made, and I wrote it down or retold it to someone else like a faithful reporter of facts, I understood that the mere act of including facts in a story did not make that story necessarily true.

A storyteller is constantly deciding: Which facts do I emphasize for importance? Which facts do I elide for simplicity? Which facts do I ignore outright because they don't fit, or because they interfere with the satisfaction of a neat ending?

But all of these questions assume there is an *I* there to do the deciding, that there is a larger underlying, never-changing, reliable fact of perspective: the fact of Me.

But now I know that this fact is a fiction.

The me who was still Me, who was tucked away somewhere behind the overwhelming pain of my spinal CSF leak, was not the me that arrived at medical appointments in a daze, everything hazy and unreal, a disconnect between my physical self and my brain, between my brain and my mouth, between my brain and my mind. It was not the me that lay on the floor, waiting, confused, unable to articulate what was happening. It was not the me that went on without me, walking without purpose, talking without thought, words racing ahead of me, meaning things I didn't intend, sounding strange to my ears, feeling foreign in my mouth.

While I was leaking, the me that was still Me was trapped inside this other me, which kept going even though I couldn't think. And yet that me was also Me, a me I wasn't aware of until the me that felt like Me was rendered incapable. Until I was able to see that the me that feels like Me is not the only me in charge of my body, my brain, my mind.

The me that feels like Me is not indisputable, not incontrovertible.

The me that feels like Me is not a fact: it is an opinion.

And if I am just an opinion my brain has formed about itself, then—even if I try to stick to the most basic facts—even the simplest story I tell is called into question due to the mystery of who, exactly, is telling it.

I am an unreliable narrator, but I'm becoming better at making sense of my story. The farther away from it I move in time, the more I'm able to understand it, place it in a context.

There are things I can't reconcile, and things I can't explain. But slowly I am coming to accept that this may be what this story is about—acknowledging the senselessness of things, accepting that things are senseless. Understanding that I can try to read my life like literature, perpetually on the lookout for foreshadowing and meaning and narrative arc; but that that won't save me or protect me from the facts, which exist even without my interpretation.

There was no warning I left unheeded, no heavy-handed metaphor I missed before the day that I coughed and tore a place inside me. I simply coughed.

I am learning how to accept this, how to explain it to myself and others. I go on dates, now, and have to account for the facts of my life, the strangeness of dating after having been married for 20 years, after a year in bed with a bizarre illness, after months of tentative recovery. It is a good litmus test: even just reciting the basic facts, without making it into a story, is enough to scare those people off who I am better off without. And the more I participate in my old life, which is simultaneously my new life—being upright, being outside, walking, remembering things, talking to people, running errands, parenting—the more I am able to consolidate the stories of the me that was Me before my leak, and the me that was Me during my leak year. This is the new Year Zero Me, slowly recovering into one single me, one single story.

I am torn between feeling betrayed by the uselessness of story and feeling grounded in the telling of it. I watch Emi move through her grief, finding her way through panic, dissociation, and anger to a place on the other side she could hardly have imagined, and I'm relieved to recognize the story arc. I watch Nate battle with anxiety, using late nights of video games and YouTube and internet to distract from his own internal windswept landscape of hyper-vigilance, eternally on the lookout for the tragedy that's already occurred, and I understand it as a kind of rite of passage.

Their story is a familiar one: the experience of a profound sense of loss as they enter the most tangled part of young adulthood and see their parents, for the first time, as flawed, separate people; the complicated, painful process of maturity as they become ever more increasingly the selves they have always been.

And mine, too, is familiar, though it's complicated in the telling: the story of illness and recovery, of living with pain, of things ending and things beginning, of learning to ask for help and also how to accept it, of finding my way back to the me that has always been Me, even though I understand now that that Me has also always been a story I told myself, a creation of my mind to make sense of my brain.

I am an unreliable narrator, most of all because I don't know how any of these stories end yet. I am like a parent telling a bedtime story in the dark, making it up as I go, hoping the sleeping selves listening are lulled by it, far too tired to be alert for discrepancies, errors, failures of the plot. But I am becoming patient with this unreliability, which I realize now has always been there, whether or not I was aware of it before. I am becoming patient with the way life defies narrative. I am becoming patient with the fact that, unreliable or not, I might not actually be the narrator at all; that I may not be the one telling the story; that the story might be telling me.

41

January 15, 2017

A year ago today, I was in a recovery room at Duke University Hospital, still drunk on a blissful mixture of Versed and fentanyl. The doctor who had just performed the procedure to seal the tear in my dura that had been causing cerebrospinal fluid to leak out of my head since March of 2015 stood over me and told me everything had gone well. "What now?" I'd asked, and Dr. Kranz had been honest. He'd told me we'd have to wait and see, that it wasn't unusual for patients to return two, three, even five or six times, for repeat procedures. "What about one time, no repeat procedures?" I'd asked, and he'd smiled. "There's always that chance," he'd said. "You could get lucky."

I'd kept smiling, but my heart sank. Because if there were such a thing as luck, surely that would have protected me from having this happen in the first place. If I were lucky, I wouldn't have been there in the recovery room, my spine like a lead pipe, the ever-present pain in my head only slightly dulled by narcotics, talking with this doctor about luck.

He'd said the 100 percent absolute best-case scenario—if I was lucky and everything went right and the CSF leak was fixed and I had no complications from the procedure and my CSF could be regulated without need for medication or draining or a shunt or repeat surgeries—was that it would take probably about a year to fully recover from the damage done to my brain.

A year.

I may not be lucky, but anyone who knows me knows that I'm fast, that I pride myself on being able to work fast; and so it's probably no surprise to learn that even in my brain-compromised state, I'd seen this as a challenge.

A year? I'd thought. *I'll do it in six months.*

I was wrong, but Dr. Kranz was right: Today it has been a year, and it has taken the full length of that year to heal.

He was also right about another thing: I got lucky.

Maybe not as lucky, in the Oscar-winning sense, as fellow CSF leaker George Clooney (who also acquired his leak in a much classier way: filming a stunt for a movie), but luckier than most people with spontaneous CSF leaks: I didn't have an underlying condition that caused this (just the unlucky convergence of a really bad flu and a really bad cough); I was diagnosed (if not treated) quickly; and I was able to get to where a team of experts were, in North Carolina, with the help of family and friends. I had setbacks during my recovery—my fall, my hospital stay, insurance woes—but none so severe that they negated my subtle but detectable progress. I was able to live off savings and book sales while I was sick, while I convalesced, while I dealt with the daily life of parenting as best I could from bed, while I navigated a divorce, while I healed. All of this was luck, I now realize, in the middle of what I thought had to be the most unlucky time of my life.

A year later I am finally beginning to take for granted once again all the things I swore I never would, from the little things, like being able to sit up and read and write, to fully participating in the world again. This is the bittersweet part of healing, the forgetting. I try to remind myself, when I realize how careless I've become, of how privileged I am to be irritated by the boringness of some simple task that would have been far too complex for me to attempt a year ago, even six months ago. I try to remind myself that this is a measure of how much healing I've done.

I try to remind myself, too, that this isn't the first time in my life I've had to start over. I had to start over as a pianist at the conservatory when my teacher had me focusing on playing just one note, relearning technique and starting at the beginning in a way that changed everything. I had to start over after being sick in college with Mystery Disease, learning how to live with pain, and then how to live beyond it. I had to start over after my time as a pianist was done, when I traded conservatory life and the study of music for working full time as an editor. I had to start over when I became a mother and my world shifted into the darkness of post-partum depression and the work of finding my way back. I had to start over when I stopped my full-time editorial job and instead took on full-time mothering and freelancing and book-writing. I had to start over after Nate's accident, which unmoored me and left me groundless. So this isn't the first time I've had to start over, not the first time I've had to engage in the process of rebuilding myself. I have had a million second acts, each one evolving out of complicated periods of pain and worry and vulnerability and acknowledgement that I didn't know exactly what to do next, and each one of them bringing me to a new, deeper understanding, of realizing that I never feel more like myself than I do when I'm in the midst of learning what I need to do and where I need to go by doing it, by going there. This spinal CSF leak, which turned into this Year Zero of recovery, which is now turning into the unknowable landscape of Year One as Post-Leak Me, has felt like something new, like something unfathomable, like something that separated me from myself. And yet I see now that Post-Leak Me is as much Me as Leak Me, and New Mom Me, and Freelance Me, and Nate's Accident Me, and Music School Me, and Sick Me.

This particular Year One is new, this is true. I haven't lived through this kind of experience yet. I don't know what the contours of this year will be, I don't know how my life will be, I don't know the shape it will take. I don't know what it's like to be healed from this brain injury, to be a single parent to my kids, to fully move on—not just yet. But I do know what it's like to be lost, to be at a loss. I do know what it's like to surrender to whatever comes next. I do know what it's like to start somewhere and get to the other side.

There is more to do, and I have further to go. I still don't know why this leak happened, if it was an accident caused by selfishness or chance or a strange quirk of my biology or by nothing at all; I don't know if it will happen again. I don't know when I'll fully be healed, if the patched place on my dura will continue to hold, if I'll need another one, if I'll ever be 100 percent cured. But I know that although I'm not all better, I'm better than I was a year ago.

As of today, that year is up. And incredibly, I'm finding myself on the other side of what turned out to be the 100 percent absolute best-case scenario. Realizing that it's safe to be right here where I am, slowly moving through time, continuing to recover. Realizing that I'm finally past the worst moments of everything so far and that I'm okay. Realizing that I'm still here, I'm still me. Torn, maybe; but not broken.

I can hardly believe my luck.

Resources

Cedars-Sinai CSF Leak Program, Cedars-Sinai Medical Center
The CSF Leak Program at the Los Angeles-based Cedars-Sinai Department of Neurosurgery provides highly specialized care to patients struggling with cerebrospinal fluid leak.

https://www.cedars-sinai.edu/Patients/Programs-and-Services /Neurosurgery/Centers-and-Programs/Cerebrospinal-Fluid-Leak/

Duke Radiology, Duke University School of Medicine, Spinal CSF Leaks
The team of interventional radiologists at the Spinal CSF Leak program at Duke University in North Carolina has revolutionized the way CSF leaks are treated.

https://radiology.duke.edu/patient-care/specialized-services /spinal-csf-leaks-2/

Spinal CSF Leak Foundation

A nonprofit health advocacy foundation dedicated to reducing the suffering of those with CSF leaks through education of the general public and health professionals; information and support of patients and caregivers; and facilitation of research.

http://spinalcsfleak.org/

CSF Leak Association

U.K.-based Scottish charitable organization working to support understanding of CSF leaks.

https://www.csfleak.info/

FOR ONLINE SUPPORT

Inspire Spinal CSF Leak Support Group and Discussion Community

Public support group.

https://www.inspire.com/groups/spinal-csf-leak/

CSF LEAKS (Cerebrospinal Fluid Leak) & Intracranial Hypotension

Public-facing page for a private Facebook group.

https://www.facebook.com/groups/31002608753/about/

National Suicide Lifeline
Free, 24/7 phone support
1-800-273-8255

https://suicidepreventionlifeline.org/

Crisis Text Line
Free, 24/7, text-based chat with crisis counselors

https://www.crisistextline.org/

Further Reading and Listening

Some of the books I read and podcasts I listened to while recovering and thinking about illness, narrative, and the brain pushed to its extremes.

BOOKS

Memoir:
Limbo: A Memoir by A. Manette Ansay
Brain on Fire: My Month of Madness by Susannah Cahalan
Wave by Sonali Deraniyagala
Tell Me Everything You Don't Remember: The Stroke That Changed My Life by Christine Hyung-Oak Lee
The Two Kinds of Decay: A Memoir by Sarah Manguso
Through the Shadowlands: A Science Writer's Odyssey Into an Illness Science Doesn't Understand by Julie Rehmeyer

Adventure:
Into the Silence: The Great War, Mallory, and the Conquest of Everest
   by Wade Davis
Terra Incognita: Travels in Antarctica by Sara Wheeler

Science and philosophy:
When Things Fall Apart: Heart Advice for Difficult Times by Pema
   Chodron
From Bacteria to Bach and Back: The Evolution of Minds by Daniel
   C. Dennett
*The Brain that Changes Itself: Stories of Personal Triumph From the
   Frontiers of Brain Science* by Norman Doidge, M.D.
*The Brain's Way of Healing: Remarkable Discoveries and Recoveries
   From the Frontiers of Neuroplasticity* by Norman Doidge, M.D.
The Trauma of Everyday Life by Mark Epstein, M.D.
*Soft-Wired: How the New Science of Brain Plasticity Can Change Your
   Life* by Michael Merzenich, Ph.D.

PODCASTS

Podcasts about brains, science, and philosophy:
10% Happier with Dan Harris
Brain Matters
Brain Science with Ginger Campbell, M.D.
Hi-Phi Nation with Dr. Barry Lam
Hidden Brain
Horizon Line
Outside Podcast
The Story Collider

Podcasts about comedy, history, language, and more:
2 Dope Queens
99% Invisible
BackStory
Crime Writers On . . .
Death, Sex & Money
Hardcore History
History Extra
How to Be Amazing
In Our Time
Invisibilia
Judge John Hodgman
Terrible, Thanks for Asking
The Hilarious World of Depression
The History of English Podcast
The Nerdist
Reply All
You Made it Weird
The Memory Palace

Acknowledgments

Writing a book can feel as lonely and isolating as an illness, but post-recovery it's clear how much support I've had along the way.

Much thanks to my many writer friends, including Mary-Kim Arnold and The Rumpus, for publishing my original piece on having a spinal CSF leak as part of their "Letters in the Mail" series; Sue O'Doherty and Rachel Simon for early discussion and encouragement as I began this project; Ann Douglas for much-needed text-based cheerleading; Ona Gritz for endless commiseration, insightful comments, and generous support throughout the writing process; and Barbara Card Atkinson, whose sharp writer's eye and wit is unmatched, and whose friendship sustains me.

Thanks to my friends, old and new, online and in person, who helped me survive my leak year, begin again in Year Zero, and emerge into Year One, including Paul Constantino, Aubrey Knight, Dresden Shumaker, Sandra Telep, and the crones of Crone Island and Themyscira. Thanks especially to Heather Ann Kaldeway and my indispensable summertime writing partner Kaitlin Costello for their early and ongoing reads of this manuscript; to Alicia Korenman, who visited me the night before my procedure at Duke and graciously hosted me when I returned to North Carolina in much better health; and to Marc Stachowski, the hospital boyfriend who became my regular boyfriend, who was able to understand me even when I literally had no words.

Thanks to the welcoming community I found in the CSF Leak Facebook group and Rebound High Pressure group, and to my "big sister" and partner in patching and recovery, Nina Pelletier, who is as funny and wise as she is supportive.

Thanks to the doctors and medical professionals who supported me through this, including Randi Platt; neurologist Abigail Chua, who pointed me in the direction of Duke; and the entire team at Duke, from Horace and Nurse Charles to PA Jeff Taylor, and most especially Dr. Peter Kranz, whose considerable expertise as a researcher and clinician in treating CSF leaks is matched only by his remarkable empathy and concern for patients. Thanks to Dr. Connie Deline, founder of the Spinal CSF Leak Foundation, for lending her time and medical expertise in reading a draft of this manuscript; and to philosopher Dr. Barry Lam, for talking to me about consciousness and the self as I began to approach this project.

Thanks to my agent, Laura Gross, who has been my cheerleader and advocate for years, and whose support mattered immensely as I began to be able to write again; and to my editor, Jessica Case, whose faith in my ability to write this book has been a privilege, and the team at Pegasus, who made the book beautiful.

Thanks to my parents, Bill and Elin Buchanan, and my sister Doe Buchanan, for their support from afar; and my sister Jessie

Buchanan for her support from up close. Thanks to Steve and Nurit Binenbaum for being there through what was a difficult period for all of us, for their generous gifts of time and of food, and for their fine grandparenting over the past almost two decades; and to Gil Binenbaum for his friendship, medical advocacy, and co-parenting. To Emi and Nate, I love you both more than you can possibly imagine. I am so lucky to be your mother.